The Definitive
DIABETIC COOKBOOK
for Beginners

Master Your Diabetes with 2000+ Days of Low-Sugar and Low-Carb Recipes, Accompanied by A 30-DAY MEAL PLAN Designed to Establish Healthy Eating Habits

Clare L. Frese

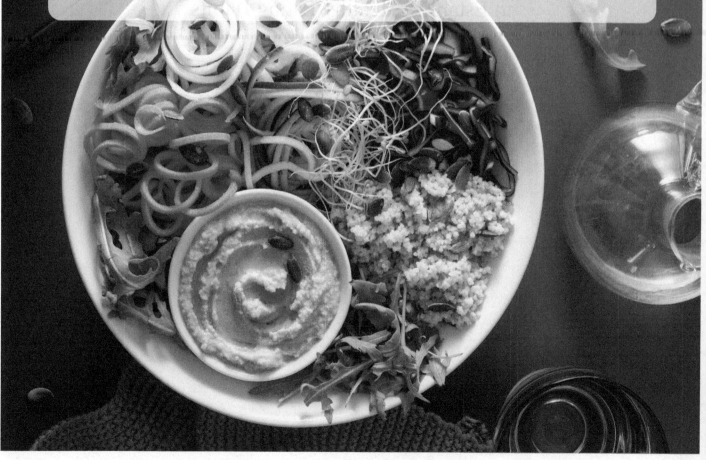

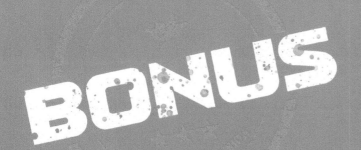

SIMPLIFY YOUR DIABETES EATING JOURNEY

2000+ Days of Low Sugar and Low Carb Diabetes Recipes

. . . .

30-Day Meal Plan to Help You Establish Healthy Eating Habits

. . . .

MANAGING DIABETES HAS NEVER BEEN EASIER!

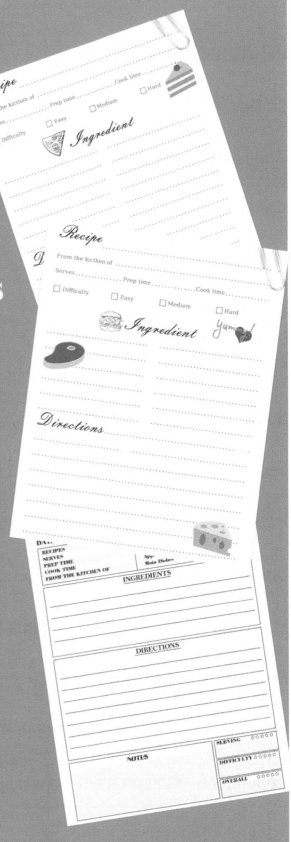

CONTENTS

INTRODUCTION 5

30-Day Meal Plan 8

Breakfast Recipes 10

Appetizers And Snacks Recipes 15

Salads Recipes 20

Vegetarian Recipes..25

Meat Recipes...30

Soups, Stews, And Chilis Recipes...35

Special Treats Recipes..40

Poultry Recipes 45

Slow Cooker Favorites Recipes 50

Potatoes, Pasta, And Whole Grains Recipes..55

Fish & Seafood Recipes..60

Vegetables, Fruit And Side Dishes Recipes...65

Appendix A: Measurement Conversions..71

Appendix B: Recipes Index 73

INTRODUCTION

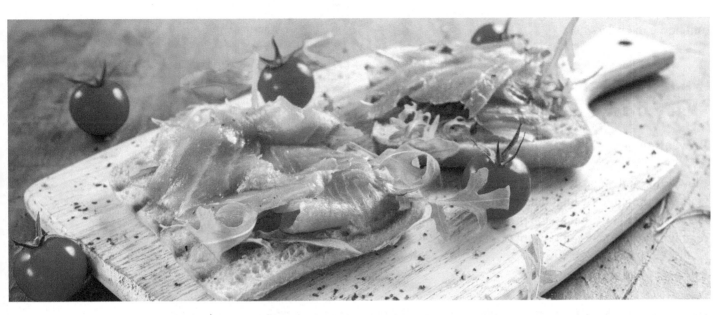

Clare L. Frese is an accomplished nutritionist, Clare has a keen understanding of diabetes, and her journey began not only in the halls of academia, but also at home as she witnessed her family's struggle with the disease. It is this personal experience, coupled with her expertise, that has led her to carefully select the recipes in this essential cookbook.

More than just a collection of recipes, Clare's The Diabetes Diet Cookbook is a statement of her belief that a diabetes diagnosis does not mean the end of delicious, satisfying meals. Instead, it's an opportunity to rediscover good food that's both healthy and enjoyable. This book is a testament to Clare's commitment to helping people with diabetes find pleasure in every bite of food while confidently managing their condition.

Flip through the book and you'll find a wide range of dishes, from hearty mains to light salads, and even some desserts that are both delicious and diabetes-friendly.

Each recipe has been carefully tailored to the needs of people with diabetes, ensuring a balanced nutritional profile and moderate carbohydrate intake. Clare's meticulous attention to detail shines through, with easy-to-follow cooking steps for each dish and an in-depth look at how each dish fits into a diabetic's diet.

The book doesn't just list ingredients and methods, though. Interspersed between the recipes is Clare's invaluable advice on controlling blood sugar levels, understanding the glycaemic index and choosing foods wisely, drawn from years of research and personal experience.

Whether you are a newly diagnosed diabetic, a long-time warrior battling diabetes, or someone looking to provide support for a loved one, Clare's Diabetic Diet Cookbook is a treasure trove of food. It is a reminder that with the right guidance and a sense of adventure, managing diabetes can be a delicious journey.

What is diabetes?

Diabetes is a chronic medical condition characterized by elevated blood sugar levels due to the body's inability to produce enough insulin or effectively use the insulin it produces. Insulin, a hormone produced by the pancreas, regulates the uptake of glucose from the bloodstream into cells for energy. There are two main types: Type 1, where the body doesn't produce insulin due to an autoimmune response, and Type 2, where the body becomes insulin resistant often due to factors like obesity and lifestyle. If not managed properly, diabetes can lead to severe health complications, including heart disease, kidney damage, and nerve disorders.

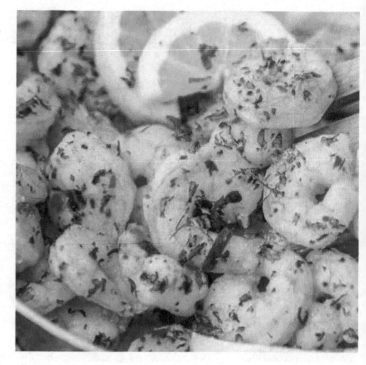

The importance of controlling blood sugar through diet

Prevention of Complications

Elevated blood sugar levels over time can lead to serious health complications, including heart disease, kidney failure, nerve damage, and vision problems. A diet that helps regulate blood sugar can prevent or delay these issues.

Energy Regulation

Blood sugar (glucose) is a primary energy source for our cells. When blood sugar levels are consistent and within a normal range, energy levels remain stable, preventing peaks of hyperactivity and crashes of fatigue.

Mood Stability

Fluctuations in blood sugar can affect mood and cognitive function. Maintaining steady blood sugar levels can help in preventing mood swings, irritability, and difficulties in concentration.

Weight Management

Diet plays a significant role in weight control. Consistently high blood sugar can lead to insulin resistance, which is linked to increased fat storage in the body. A diet that stabilizes blood sugar can aid in weight loss and prevent obesity, a significant risk factor for Type 2 diabetes.

Reduced Risk of Type 2 Diabetes

For those at risk of developing Type 2 diabetes, diet can play a preventative role. Consuming foods with a low glycemic index, which cause slower, smaller increases in blood sugar, can reduce this risk.

Improved Overall Health

Beyond diabetes, a diet that controls blood sugar typically emphasizes whole foods, lean proteins, healthy fats, and complex carbohydrates. This approach to eating promotes overall health and can prevent other chronic diseases.

In essence, the food we eat has a direct impact on blood sugar levels. Making informed dietary choices is a proactive approach to health, benefiting not just those with diabetes, but everyone striving for long-term well-being

What dietary changes can be brought about by this Diabetic Diet Cookbook?

• **Balanced Carbohydrate Intake**

The cookbook can provide recipes with calculated carbohydrate content, ensuring that each meal provides a balanced amount to avoid blood sugar spikes.

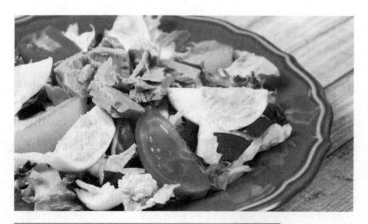

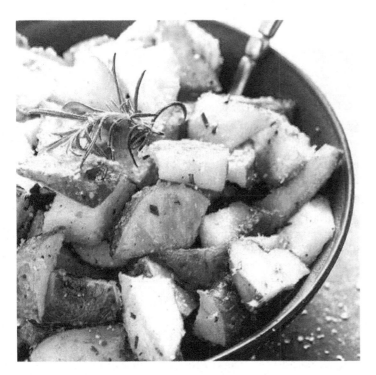

• **Low-Glycemic Foods**

Expect recipes featuring foods with a low glycemic index, which have a slower and smaller effect on blood sugar levels.

• **Inclusion of Fiber-Rich Foods**

Recipes might emphasize foods high in fiber, like legumes, vegetables, and seeds, which can help in slowing the absorption of sugar and improve blood sugar control.

• **Healthy Protein Sources**

The cookbook will likely prioritize lean protein sources like poultry, fish, tofu, and legumes, which help stabilize blood sugar levels.

• **Diverse Meal Options**

To avoid monotony, the cookbook might offer a variety of meals, from breakfasts, lunches, dinners, snacks, to desserts, all tailored to the needs of diabetics.

• **Mindful Portion Sizes**

The cookbook will likely provide guidance on portion sizes, ensuring that meals are satisfying yet within the recommended intake for maintaining healthy blood sugar levels.

Some tips for diabetics

Balanced Diet: Focus on a well-rounded diet with a mix of carbohydrates, proteins, and fats. Prioritize whole foods, lean proteins, and good fats, and minimize processed foods and those high in added sugars.

Carbohydrate Counting: Learn to count carbs. This skill is essential for insulin management and helps ensure consistent carbohydrate intake, reducing blood sugar fluctuations.

Limit Alcohol: If you drink, do so in moderation and always with food. Alcohol can affect blood sugar levels and interfere with diabetes medications.

Stay Hydrated: Drink plenty of water throughout the day. Proper hydration can help the kidneys flush out excess sugar through urine.

Avoid Smoking: Smoking increases the risk of various diabetes-related complications, including heart disease, stroke, and nerve damage. If you smoke, seek assistance in quitting.

Healthy Sleep Habits: Aim for 7-9 hours of sleep per night. Poor sleep can affect insulin sensitivity and appetite regulation.

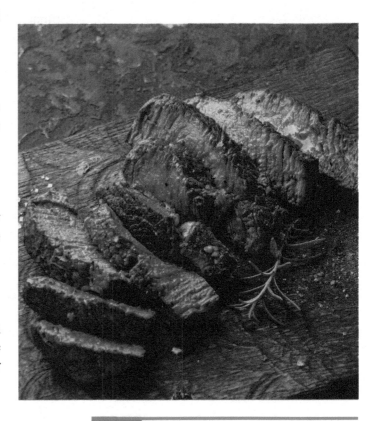

30-Day Meal Plan

Day	Breakfast	Lunch	Dinner
1	Omega-3 Granola 11	Radish, Orange, And Avocado Chopped Salad 21	Porcini-marsala Pan Sauce 31
2	Honey-yogurt Berry Salad 11	Moroccan-style Carrot Salad 21	Chard & Bacon Linguine 31
3	Maple Apple Baked Oatmeal 12	Asparagus, Red Pepper, And Spinach Salad With Goat Cheese 22	Sweet Sherry'd Pork Tenderloin 32
4	Frittata With Spinach, Bell Pepper, And Basil 12	Rainbow Veggie Salad 22	Sassy Salsa Meat Loaves 32
5	Curried Chicken Skewers With Yogurt Dipping Sauce 13	Fennel, Apple, And Chicken Chopped Salad 33	Braised Pork Stew 33
6	Double-duty Banana Pancakes 13	Zesty Citrus Melon 23	Beef En Cocotte With Mushrooms 33
7	Basil Vegetable Strata 14	Dill-marinated Broccoli 23	Stewed Beef And Ale 34
8	Sausage-egg Burritos 14	Spinach Salad With Carrots, Oranges, And Sesame 34	Grapefruit-zested Pork 34
9	Gorgonzola Polenta Bites 16	Tangy Sweet Carrot Pepper Salad 24	Spicy Tomato Pork Chops 34
10	Crostini With Kalamata Tomato 18	Bow Tie & Spinach Salad 26	Caribbean Delight 46
11	Chicken, Mango & Blue Cheese Tortillas 18	Cheese Manicotti 26	Asian Lettuce Wraps 46
12	Wicked Deviled Eggs 18	Mexican-style Spaghetti Squash Casserole 27	Oven-fried Chicken Drumsticks 47
13	Tuna Salad Stuffed Eggs 19	Stewed Chickpeas With Eggplant And Tomatoes 27	Grilled Chicken Kebabs With Tomato-feta Salad 47
14	Omega-3 Granola 11	Thai-style Red Curry With Cauliflower 28	Chicken Enchiladas 48
15	Honey-yogurt Berry Salad 11	Curried Tempeh With Cauliflower And Peas 28	Turkey Sausage Zucchini Boats 48

Day	Breakfast	Lunch	Dinner
16	Maple Apple Baked Oatmeal 12	Farro Bowl With Tofu, Mushrooms, And Spinach 29	Turkey Cutlets With Barley And Broccoli 48
17	Frittata With Spinach, Bell Pepper, And Basil 12	Tasty Lentil Tacos 29	Cumin-crusted Chicken Thighs With Cauliflower Couscous 49
18	Curried Chicken Skewers With Yogurt Dipping Sauce 13	Chickpea And Kale Soup 36	Slow Cooker Mushroom Chicken & Peas 51
19	Double-duty Banana Pancakes 13	Creamy Potato Soup With Green Onions 36	Spiced Pork Tenderloin With Carrots And Radishes 51
20	Basil Vegetable Strata 14	Salmon Dill Soup 37	Teriyaki Beef Stew 52
21	Sausage-egg Burritos 14	Shrimp Pad Thai Soup 37	Sweet Onion & Red Bell Pepper Topping 53
22	Gorgonzola Polenta Bites 16	Creamy Curried Cauliflower Soup 38	Beets With Oranges And Walnuts 53
23	Crostini With Kalamata Tomato 18	Pumpkin Turkey Chili 38	Butternut Squash With Whole Grains 53
24	Chicken, Mango & Blue Cheese Tortillas 18	Mushroom And Wheat Berry Soup 39	Pork Loin With Fennel, Oranges, And Olives 54
25	Wicked Deviled Eggs 18	Garlic-chicken And Wild Rice Soup 39	Turkey Chili 54
26	Tuna Salad Stuffed Eggs 19	Italian Cabbage Soup 52	Mustard Vinaigrette With Lemon And Parsley 61
27	Omega-3 Granola 11	Fusilli With Skillet-roasted Cauliflower, Garlic, And Walnuts 56	Crispy Fish & Chips 61
28	Honey-yogurt Berry Salad 11	Taco-spiced Rice 56	Two-sauce Cajun Fish 62
29	Maple Apple Baked Oatmeal 12	Creamy Parmesan Polenta 57	Lemon-herb Cod Fillets With Garlic Potatoes 63
30	Frittata With Spinach, Bell Pepper, And Basil 12	Warm Farro With Mushrooms And Thyme 58	Asian Snapper With Capers 63

Breakfast Recipes

Omega-3 Granola 11

Honey-yogurt Berry Salad 11

Maple Apple Baked Oatmeal 12

Frittata With Spinach, Bell Pepper, And Basil 12

Curried Chicken Skewers With Yogurt Dipping Sauce 13

Double-duty Banana Pancakes 13

Basil Vegetable Strata 14

Sausage-egg Burritos 14

Breakfast Recipes

Omega-3 Granola

Servings:6 | Cooking Time:20 Minutes

Ingredients:
- ⅓ cup slivered almonds
- ⅓ cup walnuts, chopped
- 3 cups (9 ounces) old-fashioned rolled oats
- 3 tablespoons canola oil
- ¼ cup raw sunflower seeds
- 2 tablespoons sesame seeds
- ½ cup honey
- 2 tablespoons ground flaxseeds
- ¼ teaspoon salt
- ½ cup raisins

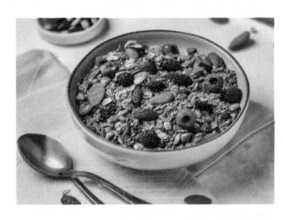

Directions:

1. Adjust oven rack to middle position and heat oven to 325 degrees. Line rimmed baking sheet with parchment paper and lightly spray with canola oil spray. Toast almonds and walnuts in 12-inch skillet over medium heat, stirring often, until fragrant and beginning to darken, about 3 minutes. Stir in oats and oil and continue to toast until oats begin to turn golden, about 2 minutes. Stir in sunflower seeds and sesame seeds and continue to toast until mixture turns golden, about 2 minutes.

2. Off heat, stir in honey, flaxseeds, and salt until well coated. Spread granola evenly over prepared sheet. Bake, stirring every few minutes, until granola is light golden brown, about 15 minutes.

3. Stir in raisins. With lightly greased stiff metal spatula, push granola onto one-half of baking sheet and press gently into ½-inch-thick slab. Let granola cool to room temperature, about 30 minutes. Loosen dried granola with spatula, break into small clusters, and serve. (Granola can be stored at room temperature in airtight container for up to 2 weeks.)

Nutrition Info:
- 240 cal., 11g fat (1g sag. fat), 0mg chol, 55mg sod., 32g carb (16g sugars, 4g fiber), 5g pro.

Honey-yogurt Berry Salad

Servings:8 | Cooking Time: 10 Minutes

Ingredients:
- 1 1/2 cups sliced fresh strawberries
- 1 1/2 cups fresh raspberries
- 1 1/2 cups fresh blueberries
- 1 1/2 cups fresh blackberries
- 1 cup (8 ounces) reduced-fat plain yogurt
- 1 tablespoon honey
- 1/4 teaspoon grated orange peel
- 1 tablespoon orange juice

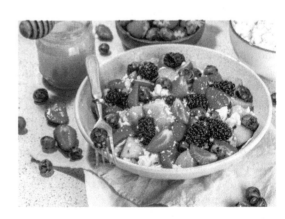

Directions:

1. Place berries in a glass bowl; toss to combine. In a small bowl, mix remaining ingredients. Spoon over berries.

Nutrition Info:
- 76 cal., 1g fat (0 sat. fat), 2mg chol., 23mg sod., 16g carb. (11g sugars, 4g fiber), 3g pro.

Maple Apple Baked Oatmeal

Servings:8 | Cooking Time: 25 Minutes

Ingredients:
- 3 cups old-fashioned oats
- 2 teaspoons baking powder
- 1 1/4 teaspoons ground cinnamon
- 1/2 teaspoon salt
- 1/4 teaspoon ground nutmeg
- 2 large eggs
- 2 cups fat-free milk
- 1/2 cup maple syrup
- 1/4 cup canola oil
- 1 teaspoon vanilla extract
- 1 large apple, chopped
- 1/4 cup sunflower kernels or pepitas

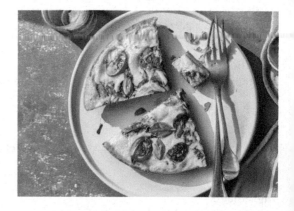

Directions:
1. Preheat oven to 350°. In a large bowl, mix the first five ingredients. In a small bowl, whisk eggs, milk, syrup, oil and vanilla until blended; stir into dry ingredients. Let stand 5 minutes. Stir in apple.
2. Transfer to an 11x7-in. baking dish coated with cooking spray. Sprinkle with sunflower kernels. Bake, uncovered, 25-30 minutes or until set and edges are lightly browned.

Nutrition Info:
- 305 cal., 13g fat (2g sat. fat), 48mg chol., 325mg sod., 41g carb. (20g sugars, 4g fiber), 8g pro.

Frittata With Spinach, Bell Pepper, And Basil

Servings:4 | Cooking Time:30minutes

Ingredients:
- 8 large eggs
- 1 ounce Parmesan cheese, grated (½ cup)
- 3 tablespoons 1 percent low-fat milk
- 2 tablespoons chopped fresh basil
- ⅛ teaspoon salt
- ¼ teaspoon pepper
- 2 teaspoons extra-virgin olive oil
- 1 small onion, chopped fine
- 1 red bell pepper, stemmed, seeded, and cut into 2-inch matchsticks
- 1 garlic clove, minced
- 3 ounces (3 cups) baby spinach

Directions:
1. Adjust oven rack to middle position and heat oven to 350 degrees. Beat eggs, Parmesan, milk, basil, salt, and pepper with fork in bowl until eggs are thoroughly combined and color is pure yellow; do not overbeat.
2. Heat oil in 10-inch ovensafe nonstick skillet over medium heat until shimmering. Add onion and bell pepper and cook until softened, about 5 minutes. Stir in garlic and cook until fragrant, about 30 seconds. Stir in spinach and cook until wilted, about 1 minute.
3. Add egg mixture and, using rubber spatula, constantly and firmly scrape along bottom and sides of skillet until eggs begin to clump and spatula just leaves trail on bottom of pan but eggs are still very wet, about 30 seconds. Smooth curds into even layer and cook, without stirring, for 30 seconds.
4. Transfer skillet to oven and bake until frittata is slightly puffy and surface is dry and bounces back when lightly pressed, 6 to 9 minutes. Run spatula around edge of skillet to loosen frittata, then carefully slide it out onto serving plate. Let sit for 5 minutes before slicing and serving.

Nutrition Info:
- 230 cal., 14g fat (4g sag. fat), 380mg chol, 370mg sod., 7g carb (3g sugars, 2g fiber), 17g pro.

Curried Chicken Skewers With Yogurt Dipping Sauce

Servings:30 | Cooking Time:1 Hou

Ingredients:
- DIPPING SAUCE
- ¾ cup low-fat plain yogurt
- ¼ cup low-fat sour cream
- 2 small garlic cloves, minced
- 3 tablespoons minced fresh mint
- 2 scallions, sliced thin
- ¼ teaspoon salt
- ⅛ teaspoon pepper
- CHICKEN
- 3 tablespoons low-fat plain yogurt
- 1 tablespoon curry powder
- ½ teaspoon salt
- ½ teaspoon paprika
- ¼ teaspoon red pepper flakes
- ¼ teaspoon garlic powder
- 2 pounds boneless, skinless chicken breasts, trimmed
- 30 (6-inch) wooden skewers
- 1 tablespoon minced fresh mint

Directions:
1. FOR THE DIPPING SAUCE Whisk all ingredients together in bowl until smooth. Cover and refrigerate until flavors meld, at least 30 minutes or up to 2 days.
2. FOR THE CHICKEN Combine yogurt, curry powder, salt, paprika, pepper flakes, and garlic powder in a large bowl. Slice chicken diagonally into ¼-inch-thick strips. Add Chicken Caesar Saladchicken to yogurt mixture and toss to coat. Cover and refrigerate for at least 1 hour or up to 24 hours.
3. Position oven rack 6 inches from broiler element and heat broiler. Set wire rack in aluminum foil–lined rimmed baking sheet and lightly spray with canola oil spray. Weave chicken onto skewers. Lay skewers on prepared rack and cover skewer ends with foil. Broil until chicken is fully cooked, 6 to 8 minutes, flipping skewers halfway through broiling. Transfer skewers to serving platter and sprinkle with mint. Serve with sauce.

Nutrition Info:
- 140 cal., 3g fat (1g sag. fat), 70mg chol, 240mg sod., 3g carb (2g sugars, 1g fiber), 22g pro.

Double-duty Banana Pancakes

Servings: 8 | Cooking Time:6 Minutes

Ingredients:
- 2 ripe medium bananas, thinly sliced
- 1 cup buckwheat pancake mix
- 3/4 cup plus 2 tablespoons fat-free milk
- 4 tablespoons light pancake syrup

Directions:
1. Mash one half of the banana slices and place in a medium bowl with the pancake mix and the milk. Stir until just blended.
2. Place a large nonstick skillet over medium heat until hot. (To test, sprinkle with a few drops of water. If the water drops "dance" or jump in the pan, it's hot enough.) Coat the skillet with nonstick cooking spray, add two scant 1/4 cup measures of batter, and cook the pancakes until puffed and dry around the edges, about 1 minute.
3. Flip the pancakes and cook until golden on the bottom. Place on a plate and cover to keep warm.
4. Recoat the skillet with nonstick cooking spray, add three scant 1/4 cup measures of batter, and cook as directed. Repeat with the remaining batter.
5. Place 2 pancakes on each of 4 dinner plates, top with equal amounts of banana slices, and drizzle evenly with the syrup. If you like, place the dinner plates in a warm oven and add the pancakes as they are cooked.

Nutrition Info:
- 100 cal., 0g fat (0g sag. fat), 0mg chol, 140mg sod., 23g carb (9g sugars, 2g fiber), 3g pro.

Basil Vegetable Strata

Servings:8 | Cooking Time: 1 Hour

Ingredients:

- 3 teaspoons canola oil, divided
- 3/4 pound sliced fresh mushrooms
- 1 cup finely chopped sweet onion
- 1 large sweet red pepper, cut into thin strips
- 1 large sweet yellow pepper, cut into thin strips
- 1 medium leek (white portion only), chopped
- 1/2 teaspoon salt
- 1/2 teaspoon pepper
- 10 slices whole wheat bread, cut into 1-inch cubes
- 1 1/2 cups shredded part-skim mozzarella cheese
- 1/4 cup grated Parmesan cheese
- 8 large eggs
- 4 large egg whites
- 2 1/2 cups fat-free milk
- 1/4 cup chopped fresh basil

Directions:

1. In a large skillet, heat 1 teaspoon oil over medium-high heat. Add the mushrooms; cook and stir 8-10 minutes or until tender. Remove from pan.
2. In same pan, heat 1 teaspoon oil over medium heat. Add onion; cook and stir 6-8 minutes or until golden brown. Add onion to mushrooms.
3. Add remaining oil to pan. Add peppers, leek, salt and pepper; cook and stir about 6-8 minutes or until leek pieces are tender. Stir in the sauteed mushrooms and onion.
4. In a 13x9-in. baking dish coated with cooking spray, layer half of each of the following: bread cubes, vegetable mixture, mozzarella cheese and Parmesan cheese. Repeat layers. In a large bowl, whisk eggs, egg whites and milk until blended; pour over layers. Sprinkle with basil. Refrigerate, covered, overnight.
5. Preheat oven to 350°. Remove the strata from refrigerator while oven heats.
6. Bake, covered, 50 minutes. Bake, uncovered, 10-15 minutes longer or until lightly browned and a knife inserted near the center comes out clean. Let strata stand 10 minutes before serving.

Nutrition Info:

- 322 cal., 13g fat (5g sat. fat), 201 mg chol., 620mg sod., 28g carb. (9g sugars, 4g fiber), 24g pro.

Sausage-egg Burritos

Servings:6 | Cooking Time: 20 Minutes

Ingredients:

- 1/2 pound bulk lean turkey breakfast sausage
- 3 large eggs
- 4 large egg whites
- 1 tablespoon olive oil
- 2 cups chopped fresh spinach
- 2 plum tomatoes, seeded and chopped
- 1 garlic clove, minced
- 1/4 teaspoon pepper
- 6 whole wheat tortillas (8 inches), warmed
- Salsa, optional

Directions:

1. In a large nonstick skillet coated with cooking spray, cook sausage over medium heat 4-6 minutes or until no longer pink, breaking into crumbles. Remove from pan.
2. In a small bowl, whisk eggs and egg whites until blended. In same pan, add eggs; cook and stir over medium heat until eggs are thickened and no liquid egg remains. Remove from pan; wipe skillet clean if necessary.
3. In a skillet, heat oil over medium-high heat. Add spinach, tomatoes and garlic; cook and stir for 2-3 minutes or until the spinach is wilted. Stir in sausage and eggs; heat through. Sprinkle mixture with pepper.
4. To serve, spoon 2/3 cup filling across center of each tortilla. Fold bottom and sides of tortilla over filling and roll up. If desired, serve with salsa.

Nutrition Info:

- 258 cal., 10g fat (2g sat. fat), 134mg chol., 596mg sod., 24g carb. (1g sugars, 4g fiber), 20g pro.

Appetizers And Snacks Recipes

Sweet Peanut Buttery Dip 16

Gorgonzola Polenta Bites 16

Mocha Pumpkin Seeds 17

Cheesy Snack Mix 17

Crostini With Kalamata Tomato 18

Chicken, Mango & Blue Cheese Tortillas 18

Wicked Deviled Eggs 18

Raisin & Hummus Pita Wedges 19

Tuna Salad Stuffed Eggs 19

Sweet Peanut Buttery Dip

Servings: 4 | Cooking Time: 5 Minutes

Ingredients:
- 1/3 cup fat-free vanilla-flavored yogurt
- 2 tablespoons reduced-fat peanut butter
- 2 teaspoons packed dark brown sugar
- 2 medium bananas, sliced

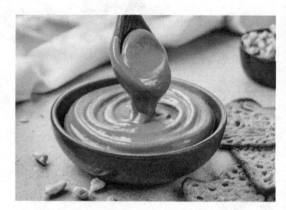

Directions:
1. Using a fork or whisk, stir the yogurt, peanut butter, and brown sugar together in a small bowl until completely blended.
2. Serve with banana slices and wooden toothpicks, if desired.

Nutrition Info:
- 120 cal., 3g fat (0g sag. fat), 0mg chol, 40mg sod., 21g carb (12g sugars, 2g fiber), 3g pro.

Gorgonzola Polenta Bites

Servings:16 | Cooking Time: 25 Minutes

Ingredients:
- 1/3 cup balsamic vinegar
- 1 tablespoon orange marmalade
- 1/2 cup panko (Japanese) bread crumbs
- 1 tube (18 ounces) polenta, cut into 16 slices
- 2 tablespoons olive oil
- 1/2 cup crumbled Gorgonzola cheese
- 3 tablespoons dried currants, optional

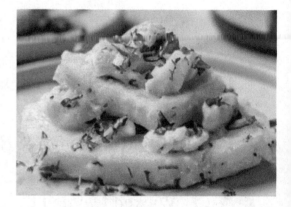

Directions:
1. In a small saucepan, combine vinegar and marmalade. Bring to a boil; cook 5-7 minutes or until liquid is reduced to 2 tablespoons.
2. Meanwhile, place bread crumbs in a shallow bowl. Press both sides of the polenta slices in bread crumbs. In a large skillet, heat oil over medium-high heat. Add polenta in batches; cook for 2-4 minutes on each side or until slices are golden brown.
3. Arrange polenta on a serving platter; spoon cheese over top. If desired, sprinkle with currants; drizzle with vinegar mixture. Serve bites warm or at room temperature.

Nutrition Info:
- 67 cal., 3g fat (1g sat. fat), 3mg chol., 161mg sod., 9g carb. (3g sugars, 0 fiber), 1g pro.

Mocha Pumpkin Seeds

Servings:3 | Cooking Time: 25 Minutes

Ingredients:
- 6 tablespoons sugar
- 2 tablespoons baking cocoa
- 1 tablespoon instant coffee granules
- 1 large egg white
- 2 cups salted shelled pumpkin seeds (pepitas)

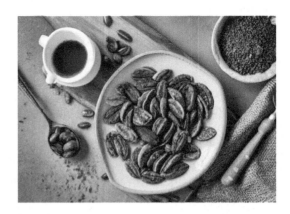

Directions:

1. Preheat oven to 325°. Place sugar, cocoa and coffee granules in a small food processor; cover and pulse until finely ground.

2. In a bowl, whisk egg white until frothy. Stir in pumpkin seeds. Sprinkle with sugar mixture; toss to coat evenly. Spread in a single layer in a parchment paper-lined 15x10x1-in. baking pan.

3. Bake 20-25 minutes or until dry and no longer sticky, stirring seeds every 10 minutes. Cool completely in pan. Store in an airtight container.

Nutrition Info:
- 142 cal., 10g fat (2g sat. fat), 0 chol., 55mg sod., 10g carb. (7g sugars, 1g fiber), 6g pro.

Cheesy Snack Mix

Servings:2 | Cooking Time: 5 Minutes

Ingredients:
- 3 cups Corn Chex
- 3 cups Rice Chex
- 3 cups cheddar miniature pretzels
- 1/4 cup butter, melted
- 1 envelope cheesy taco seasoning
- 2 cups white cheddar popcorn

Directions:

1. In a large microwave-safe bowl, combine cereal and pretzels. In a small bowl, mix melted butter and taco seasoning; drizzle over cereal mixture and toss to coat.

2. Microwave, uncovered, on high 3-3 1/2 minutes or until heated through, stirring once every minute. Stir in popcorn. Transfer to a baking sheet to cool completely. Store snack mix in an airtight container.

Nutrition Info:
- 151 cal., 5g fat (3g sat. fat), 11mg chol., 362mg sod., 23g carb. (2g sugars, 1g fiber), 3g pro.

Crostini With Kalamata Tomato

Servings: 4 | Cooking Time:10 Minutes

Ingredients:
- 4 ounces multigrain baguette bread, cut in 12 slices (about 1/4 inch thick)
- 1 small tomato, finely chopped
- 9 small kalamata olives, pitted and finely chopped
- 2 tablespoons chopped fresh basil

Directions:
1. Preheat the oven to 350°F.
2. Arrange the bread slices on a baking sheet and bake 10 minutes or until just golden on the edges. Remove from the heat and cool completely.
3. Meanwhile, stir the remaining ingredients together in a small bowl. Spread 1 tablespoon of the mixture on each bread slice.

Nutrition Info:
- 90 cal., 2g fat (0g sag. fat), 0mg chol, 220mg sod., 16g carb (2g sugars, 1g fiber), 3g pro.

Chicken, Mango & Blue Cheese Tortillas

Servings:16 | Cooking Time: 30 Minutes

Ingredients:
- 1 boneless skinless chicken breast (8 ounces)
- 1 teaspoon blackened seasoning
- 3/4 cup (6 ounces) plain yogurt
- 1 1/2 teaspoons grated lime peel
- 2 tablespoons lime juice
- 1/4 teaspoon salt
- 1/8 teaspoon pepper
- 1 cup finely chopped peeled mango
- 1/3 cup finely chopped red onion
- 4 flour tortillas (8 inches)
- 1/2 cup crumbled blue cheese
- 2 tablespoons minced fresh cilantro

Directions:
1. Lightly oil grill rack with cooking oil. Sprinkle the chicken with blackened seasoning; grill, covered, over medium heat 6-8 minutes on each side or until a thermometer reads 165°.
2. In a bowl, mix yogurt, lime peel, lime juice, salt and pepper. Cool chicken slightly; finely chop and transfer to a small bowl. Stir in mango and onion.
3. Grill tortillas, uncovered, over medium heat 2-3 minutes, until puffed. Turn; top with chicken mixture and blue cheese. Grill, covered, 2-3 minutes, until bottoms are lightly browned. Drizzle with yogurt mixture; sprinkle with cilantro. Cut each into four wedges.

Nutrition Info:
- 85 cal., 3g fat (1g sat. fat), 12mg chol., 165mg sod., 10g carb. (2g sugars, 1g fiber), 5g pro.

Wicked Deviled Eggs

Servings:2 | Cooking Time: 30 Minutes

Ingredients:
- 12 hard-cooked eggs, peeled
- 1/2 cup Miracle Whip
- 2 tablespoons cider vinegar
- 2 tablespoons prepared mustard
- 1 tablespoon minced fresh parsley or 1 teaspoon dried parsley flakes
- 1 tablespoon butter, melted
- 1 tablespoon sweet pickle relish
- 2 teaspoons Worcestershire sauce
- 1 teaspoon sweet pickle juice
- 1/2 teaspoon salt
- 1/2 teaspoon cayenne pepper
- 1/2 teaspoon pepper
- Paprika

Directions:
1. Cut eggs in half lengthwise. Remove yolks; set whites aside. In a small bowl, mash yolks. Add the Miracle Whip, vinegar, mustard, parsley, butter, relish, Worcestershire sauce, pickle juice, salt, cayenne and pepper; mix well. Stuff or pipe into egg whites.
2. Refrigerate until serving. Sprinkle with paprika.

Nutrition Info:
- 61 cal., 5g fat (1g sat. fat), 109mg chol., 151mg sod., 1g carb. (1g sugars, 0 fiber), 3g pro..

Raisin & Hummus Pita Wedges

Servings:8 | Cooking Time: 15 Minutes

Ingredients:
- 1/4 cup golden raisins
- 1 tablespoon chopped dates
- 1/2 cup boiling water
- 2 whole wheat pita breads (6 inches)
- 2/3 cup hummus
- Snipped fresh dill or dill weed, optional

Directions:
1.Place raisins and dates in a small bowl. Cover with boiling water; let stand for 5 minutes. Drain well.
2.Cut each pita into four wedges. Spread with hummus; top with raisins, dates and, if desired, dill.

Nutrition Info:
- 91 cal., 2g fat (0 sat. fat), 0 chol., 156mg sod., 16g carb. (4g sugars, 3g fiber), 3g pro.

Tuna Salad Stuffed Eggs

Servings: 4 | Cooking Time:10 Minutes

Ingredients:
- 4 large eggs
- 1 (2.6-ounce) packet tuna (or 5-ounce can of tuna packed in water, rinsed and well drained)
- 2 tablespoons reduced-fat mayonnaise
- 1 1/2–2 tablespoons sweet pickle relish

Directions:
1.Place eggs in a medium saucepan and cover with cold water. Bring to a boil over high heat, then reduce the heat and simmer 10 minutes.
2.Meanwhile, stir the tuna, mayonnaise, and relish together in a small bowl.
3.When the eggs are cooked, remove them from the water and let stand one minute before peeling under cold running water. Cut eggs in half, lengthwise, and discard 4 egg yolk halves and place the other 2 egg yolk halves in the tuna mixture and stir with a rubber spatula until well blended. Spoon equal amounts of the tuna mixture in each of the egg halves.
4.Serve immediately, or cover with plastic wrap and refrigerate up to 24 hours.

Nutrition Info:
- 90 cal., 4g fat (1g sag. fat), 105mg chol, 240mg sod., 3g carb (2g sugars, 0g fiber), 9g pro.

Salads Recipes

Radish, Orange, And Avocado Chopped Salad 21

Moroccan-style Carrot Salad 21

Asparagus, Red Pepper, And Spinach Salad With Goat Cheese 22

Rainbow Veggie Salad 22

Fennel, Apple, And Chicken Chopped Salad 23

Zesty Citrus Melon 23

Dill-marinated Broccoli 23

Spinach Salad With Carrots, Oranges, And Sesame 24

Tangy Sweet Carrot Pepper Salad 24

Salads Recipes

Radish, Orange, And Avocado Chopped Salad

Servings:6 | Cooking Time:30 Minutes

Ingredients:
- 1 cucumber, peeled, halved lengthwise, seeded, and cut into ½-inch pieces
- Salt and pepper
- 2 oranges
- 3 tablespoons extra-virgin olive oil
- 3 tablespoons lime juice (2 limes)
- 1 garlic clove, minced
- 10 radishes, trimmed, halved, and sliced thin
- ½ avocado, cut into ½-inch pieces
- ¼ cup finely chopped red onion
- 1 romaine lettuce heart (6 ounces), cut into ½-inch pieces
- 2 ounces Manchego cheese, shredded (½ cup)
- ½ cup minced fresh cilantro
- ¼ cup roasted unsalted pepitas

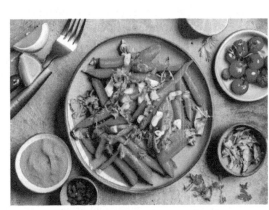

Directions:
1. Toss cucumber with ½ teaspoon salt in colander and let drain for 15 to 30 minutes.
2. Cut away peel and pith from oranges. Quarter oranges, then slice crosswise into ½-inch-thick pieces. Whisk oil, lime juice, and garlic together in large bowl. Add cucumber, orange pieces, radishes, avocado, and onion and gently toss to coat. Let sit at room temperature until flavors meld, about 5 minutes.
3. Add lettuce, Manchego, and cilantro and gently toss to coat. Season with pepper to taste and sprinkle with pepitas. Serve.

Nutrition Info:
- 200 cal., 16g fat (4g sag. fat), 5mg chol, 230mg sod., 11g carb (6g sugars, 3g fiber), 5g pro.

Moroccan-style Carrot Salad

Servings:6 | Cooking Time: 1 Hour

Ingredients:
- 2 oranges
- 1 tablespoon lemon juice
- ¾ teaspoon ground cumin
- ⅛ teaspoon cayenne pepper
- ⅛ teaspoon ground cinnamon
- Salt and pepper
- 1 pound carrots, peeled and shredded
- 3 tablespoons minced fresh cilantro
- 3 tablespoons extra-virgin olive oil

Directions:
1. Cut away peel and pith from oranges. Holding fruit over bowl, use paring knife to slice between membranes to release segments. Cut segments in half crosswise and let drain in fine-mesh strainer set over large bowl, reserving juice.
2. Whisk lemon juice, cumin, cayenne, cinnamon, and ½ teaspoon salt into bowl with reserved orange juice. Add orange segments and carrots and gently toss to coat. Let sit until liquid starts to pool in bottom of bowl, 3 to 5 minutes.
3. Drain salad in fine-mesh strainer then return to bowl. (Salad can be refrigerated for up to 1 hour; bring to room temperature before serving.) Stir in cilantro and oil and season with pepper to taste. Serve.

Nutrition Info:
- 110 cal., 7g fat (1g sag. fat), 0mg chol, 190mg sod., 12g carb (7g sugars, 3g fiber), 1g pro.

Asparagus, Red Pepper, And Spinach Salad With Goat Cheese

Servings:6 | Cooking Time:8 Minutes

Ingredients:
- 5 tablespoons extra-virgin olive oil
- 1 red bell pepper, stemmed, seeded, and cut into 2-inch-long matchsticks
- 1 pound asparagus, trimmed and cut into 1-inch lengths on bias
- Salt and pepper
- 1 shallot, sliced thin
- 1 tablespoon plus 1 teaspoon sherry vinegar
- 1 garlic clove, minced
- 6 ounces (6 cups) baby spinach
- 2 ounces goat cheese, crumbled (½ cup)

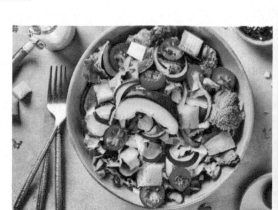

Directions:

1. Heat 1 tablespoon oil in 12-inch nonstick skillet over high heat until just smoking. Add bell pepper and cook until lightly browned, about 2 minutes. Add asparagus, ¼ teaspoon salt, and ⅛ teaspoon pepper and cook, stirring occasionally, until asparagus is browned and almost tender, about 2 minutes. Stir in shallot and cook until softened and asparagus is crisp-tender, about 1 minute. Transfer to bowl and let cool slightly.

2. Whisk remaining ¼ cup oil, vinegar, garlic, ¼ teaspoon salt, and ⅛ teaspoon pepper together in small bowl. Gently toss spinach with 2 tablespoons dressing until coated. Season with pepper to taste. Divide spinach among individual plates. Gently toss asparagus mixture with remaining dressing and arrange over spinach. Sprinkle with goat cheese. Serve.

Nutrition Info:
- 160 cal., 14g fat (3g sag. fat), 5mg chol, 260mg sod., 6g carb (3g sugars, 3g fiber), 4g pro.

Rainbow Veggie Salad

Servings:8 | Cooking Time: 25 Minutes

Ingredients:
- 1/2 English cucumber, cut lengthwise in half and sliced
- 2 medium carrots, thinly sliced
- 1 cup each red and yellow cherry tomatoes, halved
- 3/4 cup pitted ripe olives, halved
- 1 celery rib, thinly sliced
- 1/4 cup each chopped sweet yellow, orange and red pepper
- 1/4 cup thinly sliced red onion
- 1/8 teaspoon garlic salt
- Dash coarsely ground pepper
- 1 package (5 ounces) spring mix salad greens
- 2/3 cup reduced-fat buttermilk ranch salad dressing

Directions:

1. Place cucumber, carrots, tomatoes, olives, celery, sweet peppers, onion, garlic salt and pepper in a large bowl; toss to combine.

2. Just before serving, add salad greens. Drizzle with dressing and toss gently to combine.

Nutrition Info:
- 64 cal., 3g fat (1g sat. fat), 0 chol., 232mg sod., 7g carb. (3g sugars, 2g fiber), 2g pro.

Fennel, Apple, And Chicken Chopped Salad

Servings:4 | Cooking Time:75 Minutes

Ingredients:
- 1 cucumber, peeled, halved lengthwise, seeded, and sliced ½ inch thick
- Salt and pepper
- 1 pound boneless, skinless chicken breasts, trimmed of all visible fat and pounded to ¾-inch thickness
- 3 ounces goat cheese, crumbled (¾ cup)
- ¼ cup cider vinegar
- ¼ cup minced fresh tarragon
- 1 tablespoon extra-virgin olive oil
- 2 Fuji, Gala, or Golden Delicious apples, cored, quartered, and sliced crosswise ¼ inch thick
- 1 fennel bulb, stalks discarded, bulb halved, cored, and sliced ¼ inch thick
- ½ cup finely chopped red onion
- 1 romaine lettuce heart (6 ounces), cut into ½-inch pieces

Directions:
1. Toss cucumber with ½ teaspoon salt in colander and let drain for 15 to 30 minutes.
2. Whisk 4 quarts water and 2 tablespoons salt in Dutch oven until salt is dissolved. Arrange breasts, skinned side up, in steamer basket, making sure not to overlap them. Submerge steamer basket in water.
3. Heat pot over medium heat, stirring liquid occasionally to even out hot spots, until water registers 175 degrees, 15 to 20 minutes. Turn off heat, cover pot, remove from burner, and let sit until meat registers 160 degrees, 17 to 22 minutes. Transfer chicken to paper towel–lined plate and refrigerate until cool, about 30 minutes. (Chicken can be refrigerated for up to 2 days.)
4. Whisk goat cheese, vinegar, tarragon, and oil together in large bowl. Pat chicken dry with paper towels and cut into ½-inch pieces. Add chicken, cucumber, apples, fennel, and onion to dressing and gently toss to coat. Let sit at room temperature until flavors meld, about 5 minutes. Add lettuce and gently toss to coat. Season with pepper to taste. Serve.

Nutrition Info:
- 310 cal., 11g fat (4g sag. fat), 95mg chol, 410mg sod., 22g carb (14g sugars, 5g fiber), 32g pro.

Zesty Citrus Melon

Servings: 4 | Cooking Time: 5 Minutes

Ingredients:
- 1/4 cup orange juice
- 2–3 tablespoons lemon juice
- 1 teaspoon honey
- 3 cups diced honeydew or cantaloupe melon

Directions:
1. Stir the orange juice, lemon zest (if using), lemon juice, and honey together in a small bowl.
2. Place the melon on a serving plate and pour the juice mixture evenly over all. For peak flavor, serve within 1 hour.

Nutrition Info:
- 60 cal., 0g fat (0g sag. fat), 0mg chol, 25mg sod., 15g carb (13g sugars, 1g fiber), 1g pro.

Dill-marinated Broccoli

Servings:8 | Cooking Time: 15 Minutes

Ingredients:
- 6 cups fresh broccoli florets
- 1 cup canola oil
- 1 cup cider vinegar
- 2 tablespoons snipped fresh dill
- 2 teaspoons sugar
- 1 teaspoon garlic salt
- 1 teaspoon salt

Directions:
1. Place broccoli in a large resealable plastic bag. Whisk together remaining ingredients; add to broccoli. Seal bag and turn to coat; refrigerate 4 hours or overnight. To serve, drain broccoli, discarding marinade.

Nutrition Info:
- 79 cal., 7g fat (1g sat. fat), 0 chol., 119mg sod., 3g carb. (0 sugars, 2g fiber), 2g pro.

Spinach Salad With Carrots, Oranges, And Sesame

Servings:6 | Cooking Time:15 Minutes

Ingredients:
- 2 oranges
- 2 carrots, peeled
- 2 tablespoons rice vinegar
- 1 small shallot, minced
- 1 teaspoon Dijon mustard
- ¾ teaspoon mayonnaise
- ⅛ teaspoon salt
- 2½ tablespoons canola oil
- ¾ teaspoon toasted sesame oil
- 6 ounces (6 cups) baby spinach
- 2 scallions, sliced thin
- 1½ teaspoons toasted sesame seeds

Directions:
1. Grate ½ teaspoon zest from 1 orange; set zest aside. Cut away peel and pith from oranges. Holding fruit over fine-mesh strainer set in bowl, use paring knife to slice between membranes to release segments. Measure out and reserve 2 tablespoons juice; discard remaining juice. Using vegetable peeler, shave carrots lengthwise into ribbons.
2. Whisk orange zest and reserved juice, vinegar, shallot, mustard, mayonnaise, and salt together in large bowl. While whisking constantly, drizzle in oils until completely emulsified. Add orange segments, carrots, spinach, and scallions and gently toss to coat. Sprinkle with sesame seeds. Serve.

Nutrition Info:
- 110 cal., 7g fat (0g sag. fat), 0mg chol, 110mg sod., 10g carb (5g sugars, 3g fiber), 2g pro.

Tangy Sweet Carrot Pepper Salad

Servings: 4 | Cooking Time:1 Minute

Ingredients:
- 1 1/2 cups peeled sliced carrots (about 1/8-inch thick)
- 2 tablespoons water
- 3/4 cup thinly sliced green bell pepper
- 1/3 cup thinly sliced onion
- 1/4 cup reduced-fat Catalina dressing

Directions:
1. Place carrots and water in a shallow, microwave-safe dish, such as a glass pie plate. Cover with plastic wrap and microwave on HIGH for 1 minute or until carrots are just tender-crisp. Be careful not to overcook them—the carrots should retain some crispness.
2. Immediately place the carrots in a colander and run under cold water about 30 seconds to cool. Shake to drain and place the carrots on paper towels to dry further. Dry the dish.
3. When the carrots are completely cool, return them to the dish, add the remaining ingredients, and toss gently to coat.
4. Serve immediately, or chill 30 minutes for a more blended flavor. Flavors are at their peak if you serve this salad within 30 minutes of adding dressing.

Nutrition Info:
- 60 cal., 0g fat (0g sag. fat), 0mg chol, 200mg sod., 11g carb (7g sugars, 2g fiber), 1g pro.

Vegetarian Recipes

Bow Tie & Spinach Salad...26

Cheese Manicotti...26

Mexican-style Spaghetti Squash Casserole....................................27

Stewed Chickpeas With Eggplant And Tomatoes...........................27

Thai-style Red Curry With Cauliflower...28

Curried Tempeh With Cauliflower And Peas...................................28

Farro Bowl With Tofu, Mushrooms, And Spinach...........................29

Tasty Lentil Tacos..29

Vegetarian Recipes

Bow Tie & Spinach Salad

Servings:6 | Cooking Time: 30 Minutes

Ingredients:
- 2 cups uncooked multigrain bow tie pasta
- 1 can (15 ounces) chickpeas, rinsed and drained
- 6 cups fresh baby spinach (about 6 ounces)
- 2 cups fresh broccoli florets
- 2 plum tomatoes, chopped
- 1 medium sweet red pepper, chopped
- 1/2 cup cubed part-skim mozzarella cheese
- 1/2 cup pitted Greek olives, halved
- 1/4 cup minced fresh basil
- 1/3 cup reduced-fat sun-dried tomato salad dressing
- 1/4 teaspoon salt
- 1/4 cup chopped walnuts, toasted

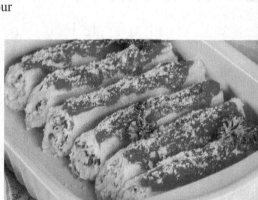

Directions:
1. Cook pasta according to package directions. Drain; transfer to a bowl.
2. Add beans, vegetables, cheese, olives and basil to pasta. Drizzle with dressing and sprinkle with salt; toss to coat. Sprinkle with walnuts.

Nutrition Info:
- 319 cal., 13g fat (2g sat. fat), 6mg chol., 660mg sod., 39g carb. (6g sugars, 7g fiber), 14g pro.

Cheese Manicotti

Servings:7 | Cooking Time: 1 Hour

Ingredients:
- 1 carton (15 ounces) reduced-fat ricotta cheese
- 1/2 cup shredded part-skim mozzarella cheese
- 1 small onion, finely chopped
- 1 large egg, lightly beaten
- 2 tablespoons minced fresh parsley
- 1/2 teaspoon pepper
- 1/4 teaspoon salt
- 1 cup grated Parmesan cheese, divided
- 4 cups marinara sauce
- 1/2 cup water
- 1 package (8 ounces) manicotti shells

Directions:
1. Preheat oven to 350°. In a small bowl, mix the first seven ingredients; stir in 1/2 cup Parmesan cheese. In another bowl, mix marinara sauce and water; spread 3/4 cup sauce onto bottom of a 13x9-in. baking dish coated with cooking spray. Fill uncooked manicotti shells with ricotta mixture; arrange over sauce. Top with remaining sauce.
2. Bake, covered, 50 minutes or until pasta is tender. Sprinkle with remaining Parmesan cheese. Bake, uncovered, 10-15 minutes longer or until the cheese is melted.

Nutrition Info:
- 340 cal., 8g fat (5g sat. fat), 60mg chol., 615mg sod., 46g carb. (16g sugars, 4g fiber), 19g pro.

Mexican-style Spaghetti Squash Casserole

Servings:4 | Cooking Time:45 Minutes

Ingredients:
- 1 (2½- to 3-pound) spaghetti squash, halved lengthwise and seeded
- 3 tablespoons extra-virgin olive oil
- Salt and pepper
- 2 garlic cloves, minced
- ½ teaspoon smoked paprika
- ½ teaspoon ground cumin
- 1 (15-ounce) can no-salt-added black beans, rinsed
- 1 cup frozen corn
- 6 ounces cherry tomatoes, quartered
- 6 scallions (4 minced, 2 sliced thin)
- 1 jalapeño chile, stemmed, seeded, and minced
- 1 avocado, halved, pitted, and cut into ½-inch pieces
- 2 ounces queso fresco, crumbled (½ cup)
- Lime wedges

Directions:
1. Adjust oven rack to middle position and heat oven to 375 degrees. Lightly spray 8-inch square baking dish with vegetable oil spray. Brush cut sides of squash with 1 tablespoon oil and sprinkle with ⅛ teaspoon salt and ¼ teaspoon pepper. Place squash cut side down in prepared dish (squash will not sit flat in dish) and roast until just tender, 40 to 45 minutes. Flip squash cut side up and let sit until cool enough to handle, about 20 minutes. Do not turn off oven.
2. Combine remaining 2 tablespoons oil, garlic, paprika, cumin, and ½ teaspoon salt in large bowl and microwave until fragrant, about 30 seconds. Stir in beans, corn, tomatoes, minced scallions, and jalapeño.
3. Using fork, scrape squash into strands in bowl with bean mixture. Stir to combine, then spread mixture evenly in now-empty dish and cover tightly with aluminum foil. Bake until heated through, 20 to 25 minutes. Sprinkle with avocado, queso fresco, and sliced scallions. Serve with lime wedges.

Nutrition Info:
- 400 cal., 24g fat (4g sag. fat), 10mg chol, 520mg sod., 41g carb (9g sugars, 11g fiber), 11g pro.

Stewed Chickpeas With Eggplant And Tomatoes

Servings:6 | Cooking Time: 60 Minutes

Ingredients:
- ¼ cup extra-virgin olive oil
- 2 onions, chopped
- 1 green bell pepper, stemmed, seeded, and chopped fine
- Salt and pepper
- 3 garlic cloves, minced
- 1 tablespoon minced fresh oregano or 1 teaspoon dried
- 2 bay leaves
- 1 pound eggplant, cut into 1-inch pieces
- 1 (28-ounce) can no-salt-added whole peeled tomatoes, drained with juice reserved, chopped coarse
- 2 (15-ounce) cans no-salt-added chickpeas, drained with 1 cup liquid reserved

Directions:
1. Adjust oven rack to lower-middle position and heat oven to 400 degrees. Heat oil in Dutch oven over medium heat until shimmering. Add onions, bell pepper, ½ teaspoon salt, and ¼ teaspoon pepper and cook until softened, about 5 minutes. Stir in garlic, 1 teaspoon oregano, and bay leaves and cook until fragrant, about 30 seconds.
2. Stir in eggplant, tomatoes and reserved juice, and chickpeas and reserved liquid and bring to boil. Transfer pot to oven and cook, uncovered, until eggplant is very tender, 45 to 60 minutes, stirring twice during cooking.
3. Discard bay leaves. Stir in remaining 2 teaspoons oregano and season with pepper to taste. Serve.

Nutrition Info:
- 270 cal., 10g fat (1g sag. fat), 0mg chol, 470mg sod., 34g carb (9g sugars, 9g fiber), 9g pro.

Thai-style Red Curry With Cauliflower

Servings:4 | Cooking Time:10 Minutes

Ingredients:
- 1 (13.5-ounce) can light coconut milk
- 1 tablespoon fish sauce
- 1 teaspoon grated lime zest plus 1 tablespoon juice
- 2 teaspoons Thai red curry paste
- ⅛ teaspoon red pepper flakes
- 2 tablespoons plus 1 teaspoon canola oil
- 2 garlic cloves, minced
- 1 teaspoon grated fresh ginger
- 1 large head cauliflower (3 pounds), cored and cut into ¾-inch florets
- ¼ cup fresh basil leaves, torn into rough ½-inch pieces

Directions:
1. Whisk coconut milk, fish sauce, lime zest and juice, curry paste, and pepper flakes together in bowl. In separate bowl, combine 1 teaspoon oil, garlic, and ginger.
2. Heat remaining 2 tablespoons oil in 12-inch nonstick skillet over high heat until shimmering. Add cauliflower and ¼ cup water, cover, and cook until cauliflower is just tender and translucent, about 5 minutes. Uncover and continue to cook, stirring occasionally, until liquid is evaporated and cauliflower is tender and well browned, 8 to 10 minutes.
3. Push cauliflower to sides of skillet. Add garlic mixture and cook, mashing mixture into skillet, until fragrant, about 30 seconds. Stir garlic mixture into cauliflower and reduce heat to medium-high. Whisk coconut milk mixture to recombine, add to skillet, and simmer until slightly thickened, about 4 minutes. Off heat, stir in basil. Serve.

Nutrition Info:
- 200 cal., 13g fat (4g sag. fat), 0mg chol, 380mg sod., 20g carb (7g sugars, 7g fiber), 7g pro.

Curried Tempeh With Cauliflower And Peas

Servings:6 | Cooking Time:15 Minutes

Ingredients:
- 1 (14.5-ounce) no-salt-added can diced tomatoes
- ¼ cup canola oil
- 2 tablespoons curry powder
- 1½ teaspoons garam masala
- 2 onions, chopped fine
- Salt and pepper
- 3 garlic cloves, minced
- 1 tablespoon grated fresh ginger
- 1 serrano chile, stemmed, seeded, and minced
- 1 tablespoon no-salt-added tomato paste
- ½ head cauliflower (1 pound), cored and cut into 1-inch florets
- 8 ounces tempeh, cut into 1-inch pieces
- 1¼ cups water
- 1 cup frozen peas
- ¼ cup light coconut milk
- 2 tablespoons minced fresh cilantro
- Lime wedges

Directions:
1. Pulse diced tomatoes with their juice in food processor until nearly smooth, with some ¼-inch pieces visible, about 3 pulses.
2. Heat oil in Dutch oven over medium-high heat until shimmering. Add curry powder and garam masala and cook until fragrant, about 10 seconds. Add onions and ¼ teaspoon salt and cook, stirring occasionally, until softened and browned, about 10 minutes.
3. Reduce heat to medium. Stir in garlic, ginger, serrano, and tomato paste and cook until fragrant, about 30 seconds. Add cauliflower and tempeh and cook, stirring constantly, until florets are coated with spices, about 2 minutes.
4. Gradually stir in water, scraping up any browned bits. Stir in tomatoes and bring to simmer. Cover, reduce heat to low, and cook until vegetables are tender, 10 to 15 minutes.
5. Stir in peas, coconut milk, and ¾ teaspoon salt and cook until heated through, 1 to 2 minutes. Off heat, stir in cilantro and season with pepper to taste. Serve with lime wedges.

Nutrition Info:
- 240 cal., 15g fat (2g sag. fat), 0mg chol, 430mg sod., 19g carb (6g sugars, 6g fiber), 12g pro.

Farro Bowl With Tofu, Mushrooms, And Spinach

Servings:4 | Cooking Time:30 Minutes

Ingredients:

- 2 tablespoons mayonnaise
- 5 teaspoons toasted sesame oil
- 1 tablespoon red miso
- 2 teaspoons sherry vinegar
- 1 teaspoon grated fresh ginger
- 1 cup whole farro
- Salt
- 14 ounces firm tofu
- 3 tablespoons cornstarch
- ¼ cup canola oil
- 10 ounces cremini mushrooms, trimmed and chopped coarse
- 2 tablespoons dry sherry
- 10 ounces (10 cups) baby spinach
- 2 scallions, sliced thin

Directions:

1. Whisk mayonnaise, 1 tablespoon sesame oil, miso, 1 tablespoon water, 1 teaspoon vinegar, and ginger together in small bowl; set sauce aside for serving.
2. Bring 4 quarts water to boil in large pot. Add farro and 1 teaspoon salt and cook until grains are tender with slight chew, 15 to 30 minutes. Drain farro well and return to now-empty pot. Stir in remaining 2 teaspoons sesame oil and remaining 1 teaspoon vinegar and cover to keep warm.
3. Meanwhile, cut tofu crosswise into 8 equal slabs, arrange over paper towel–lined baking sheet, and let drain for 20 minutes. Gently press dry with paper towels.
4. Spread cornstarch in shallow dish. Coat tofu thoroughly in cornstarch, pressing gently to adhere; transfer to plate. Heat 2 tablespoons canola oil in 12-inch nonstick skillet over medium-high heat until just smoking. Add tofu and cook until crisp and browned, about 4 minutes per side. Transfer to paper towel–lined plate and tent with aluminum foil. Wipe skillet clean with paper towels.
5. Heat 1 tablespoon canola oil in now-empty skillet over medium-high heat until shimmering. Add mushrooms and ⅛ teaspoon salt and cook until beginning to brown, 5 to 8 minutes. Stir in sherry and cook, scraping up any browned bits, until skillet is nearly dry, about 1 minute; transfer to bowl.
6. Heat remaining 1 tablespoon canola oil in again-empty skillet over medium-high heat until shimmering. Add spinach, 1 handful at a time, and cook until just wilted, about 1 minute. Divide farro among individual serving bowls, then top with tofu, mushrooms, and spinach. Drizzle with miso-ginger sauce, sprinkle with scallions, and serve.

Nutrition Info:

- 530 cal., 31g fat (3g sag. fat), 5mg chol, 420mg sod., 48g carb (5g sugars, 7g fiber), 18g pro.

Tasty Lentil Tacos

Servings:6 | Cooking Time: 40 Minutes

Ingredients:

- 1 teaspoon canola oil
- 1 medium onion, finely chopped
- 1 garlic clove, minced
- 1 cup dried lentils, rinsed
- 1 tablespoon chili powder
- 2 teaspoons ground cumin
- 1 teaspoon dried oregano
- 2 1/2 cups vegetable or reduced-sodium chicken broth
- 1 cup salsa
- 12 taco shells
- 1 1/2 cups shredded lettuce
- 1 cup chopped fresh tomatoes
- 1 1/2 cups shredded reduced-fat cheddar cheese
- 6 tablespoons fat-free sour cream

Directions:

1. In a large nonstick skillet, heat oil over medium heat; saute onion and garlic until tender. Add the lentils and seasonings; cook and stir 1 minute. Stir in broth; bring to a boil. Reduce heat; simmer, covered, until lentils are tender, 25-30 minutes.
2. Cook, uncovered, until mixture is thickened, for 6-8 minutes, stirring occasionally. Mash lentils slightly; stir in salsa and heat through. Serve in taco shells. Top with remaining ingredients.

Nutrition Info:

- 365 cal., 12g fat (5g sat. fat), 21mg chol., 777mg sod., 44g carb. (5g sugars, 6g fiber), 19g pro.

Meat Recipes

Porcini-marsala Pan Sauce 31

Chard & Bacon Linguine 31

Sweet Sherry'd Pork Tenderloin 32

Sassy Salsa Meat Loaves 32

Braised Pork Stew 33

Beef En Cocotte With Mushrooms 33

Stewed Beef And Ale 34

Grapefruit-zested Pork 34

Spicy Tomato Pork Chops 34

Meat Recipes

Porcini-marsala Pan Sauce

Servings:4 | Cooking Time:30 Seconds

Ingredients:
- This recipe is meant to be started after you have seared steak or chicken in a skillet. Do not wash the skillet after searing—any remaining browned bits add important flavor to the sauce.
- ¾ cup unsalted chicken broth
- ¼ ounce dried porcini mushrooms, rinsed
- 1 shallot, minced
- ½ cup dry Marsala
- 2 tablespoons unsalted butter, cut into 2 pieces and chilled
- 1 tablespoon minced fresh parsley
- Pepper

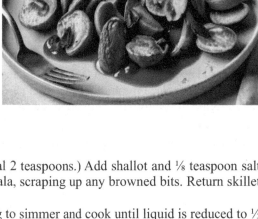

Directions:
1. Microwave ½ cup broth and mushrooms in covered bowl until steaming, about 1 minute. Let sit until softened, about 5 minutes. Drain mushrooms through fine-mesh strainer lined with coffee filter, reserving soaking liquid, and finely chop mushrooms.
2. Pour off all but 2 teaspoons fat from skillet. (Or, if necessary, add oil to equal 2 teaspoons.) Add shallot and ⅛ teaspoon salt and cook over medium heat until softened, 1 to 2 minutes. Off heat, stir in Marsala, scraping up any browned bits. Return skillet to medium heat and simmer until Marsala is reduced to glaze, about 3 minutes.
3. Stir in remaining ¼ cup broth, reserved soaking liquid, and mushrooms. Bring to simmer and cook until liquid is reduced to ⅓ cup, 4 to 6 minutes. Off heat, whisk in butter, 1 piece at a time, until combined, then whisk in parsley and any accumulated meat juices. Season with pepper to taste. Serve immediately.

Nutrition Info:
- 110 cal., 6g fat (3g sag. fat), 15mg chol, 220mg sod., 6g carb (5g sugars, 1g fiber), 2g pro.

Chard & Bacon Linguine

Servings:4 | Cooking Time: 30 Minutes

Ingredients:
- 8 ounces uncooked whole wheat linguine
- 4 bacon strips, chopped
- 4 garlic cloves, minced
- 1/2 cup reduced-sodium chicken broth
- 1/2 cup dry white wine or additional chicken broth
- 1/4 teaspoon salt
- 6 cups chopped Swiss chard (about 6 ounces)
- 1/3 cup shredded Parmesan cheese

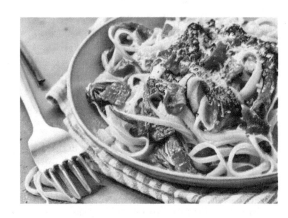

Directions:
1. Cook linguine according to package directions; drain. Meanwhile, in a large skillet, cook bacon over medium heat until crisp, stirring occasionally. Add garlic; cook 1 minute longer.
2. Add the broth, wine, salt and Swiss chard to skillet; bring to a boil. Cook and stir 4-5 minutes or until chard is tender.
3. Add linguine; heat through, tossing to combine. Sprinkle with cheese.

Nutrition Info:
- 353 cal., 14g fat (5g sat. fat), 23mg chol., 633mg sod., 47g carb. (2g sugars, 7g fiber), 14g pro.

Sweet Sherry'd Pork Tenderloin

Servings: 4 | Cooking Time:22 Minutes

Ingredients:
- 1 pound pork tenderloin
- 1/4 cup dry sherry (divided use)
- 3 tablespoons lite soy sauce (divided use)
- 1/3 cup peach all-fruit spread

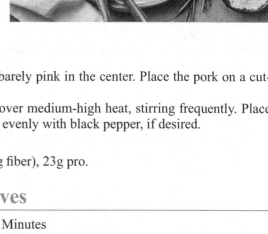

Directions:

1. Place the pork, 2 tablespoons sherry, and 2 tablespoons soy sauce in a quart-sized zippered plastic bag. Seal tightly and toss back and forth to coat evenly. Refrigerate overnight or at least 8 hours.

2. Stir the fruit spread, 2 tablespoons sherry, and 1 tablespoon soy sauce together in a small bowl. Cover with plastic wrap and refrigerate until needed.

3. Preheat the oven to 425°F.

4. Remove the pork from the marinade and discard the marinade. Place a medium nonstick skillet over medium-high heat until hot. Coat the skillet with nonstick cooking spray, add the pork, and brown on all sides.

5. Place the pork in a 9-inch pie pan and bake 15 minutes or until the pork is barely pink in the center. Place the pork on a cutting board and let stand 3 minutes before slicing.

6. Meanwhile, place the fruit spread mixture in the skillet and bring to a boil over medium-high heat, stirring frequently. Place the sauce on the bottom of a serving plate and arrange the pork on top. Sprinkle evenly with black pepper, if desired.

Nutrition Info:
- 190 cal., 3g fat (1g sag. fat), 60mg chol, 320mg sod., 14g carb (11g sugars, 0g fiber), 23g pro.

Sassy Salsa Meat Loaves

Servings:2 | Cooking Time: 1 Hour 5 Minutes

Ingredients:
- 3/4 cup uncooked instant brown rice
- 1 can (8 ounces) tomato sauce
- 1 1/2 cups salsa, divided
- 1 large onion, chopped
- 1 large egg, lightly beaten
- 1 celery rib, finely chopped
- 1/4 cup minced fresh parsley
- 2 tablespoons minced fresh cilantro
- 2 garlic cloves, minced
- 1 tablespoon chili powder
- 1 1/2 teaspoons salt
- 1/2 teaspoon pepper
- 2 pounds lean ground beef (90% lean)
- 1 pound ground turkey
- 1/2 cup shredded reduced-fat Monterey Jack cheese or Mexican cheese blend

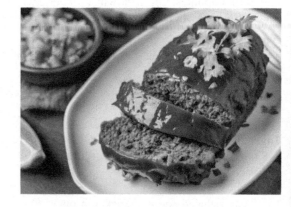

Directions:

1. Preheat oven to 350°. Cook rice according to package directions; cool slightly. In a large bowl, combine tomato sauce, 1/2 cup salsa, onion, egg, celery, parsley, cilantro, garlic and seasonings; stir in rice. Add beef and turkey; mix lightly but thoroughly.

2. Shape into two 8x4-in. loaves on a greased rack in a broiler pan. Bake 1 to 1 1/4 hours or until a meat thermometer reads 165°.

3. Spread with remaining salsa; sprinkle with cheese; bake 5 minutes or until cheese is melted. Let stand 10 minutes before slicing.

Nutrition Info:
- 237 cal., 11g fat (4g sat. fat), 91mg chol., 634mg sod., 9g carb. (2g sugars, 1g fiber), 25g pro.

Braised Pork Stew

Servings:4 | Cooking Time: 30 Minutes

Ingredients:
- 1 pound pork tenderloin, cut into 1-inch cubes
- 1/2 teaspoon salt
- 1/2 teaspoon pepper
- 5 tablespoons all-purpose flour, divided
- 1 tablespoon olive oil
- 1 package (16 ounces) frozen vegetables for stew
- 1 1/2 cups reduced-sodium chicken broth
- 2 garlic cloves, minced
- 2 teaspoons stone-ground mustard
- 1 teaspoon dried thyme
- 2 tablespoons water

Directions:
1. Sprinkle pork with salt and pepper; add 3 tablespoons flour and toss to coat. In a large skillet, heat oil over medium heat. Brown pork. Drain if necessary. Stir in vegetables, broth, garlic, mustard and thyme. Bring to a boil. Reduce heat; simmer, covered, for 10-15 minutes or until pork and vegetables are tender.
2. In a small bowl, mix remaining flour and water until smooth; stir into stew. Return to a boil, stirring constantly; cook and stir 1-2 minutes or until stew is thickened.

Nutrition Info:
- 275 cal., 8g fat (2g sat. fat), 63mg chol., 671mg sod., 24g carb. (2g sugars, 1g fiber), 26g pro.

Beef En Cocotte With Mushrooms

Servings:12 | Cooking Time:20 Minutes

Ingredients:
- 1 (3-pound) top sirloin roast, trimmed of all visible fat and tied at 1½-inch intervals
- Salt and pepper
- 4 teaspoons canola oil
- 8 ounces cremini mushrooms, trimmed and sliced thin
- 1 onion, halved and sliced thin
- ½ ounce dried porcini mushrooms, rinsed and minced
- 6 garlic cloves, lightly crushed and peeled
- 1 tablespoon no-salt added tomato paste
- ¼ cup dry white wine
- 2 tablespoons cognac
- 2 sprigs fresh tarragon, plus 2 tablespoons minced
- 2 cups unsalted chicken broth

Directions:
1. Adjust oven rack to lowest position and heat oven to 250 degrees. Pat roast dry with paper towels and sprinkle with ¾ teaspoon salt and ½ teaspoon pepper. Heat 2 teaspoons oil in Dutch oven over medium-high heat until just smoking. Brown beef on all sides, about 10 minutes; transfer to plate.
2. Add cremini mushrooms, onion, porcini mushrooms, and remaining 2 teaspoons oil to fat left in pot. Cover and cook until mushrooms release their moisture, about 5 minutes. Uncover and continue to cook, stirring often, until liquid has evaporated and vegetables are well browned, 5 to 7 minutes.
3. Stir in garlic and tomato paste and cook until fragrant, about 30 seconds. Stir in wine and cognac, scraping up any browned bits, and cook until nearly evaporated, about 1 minute. Add tarragon sprigs.
4. Nestle roast into pot along with any accumulated juices. Place large sheet of aluminum foil over pot and press to seal, then cover tightly with lid. Transfer pot to oven and cook until meat registers 120 to 125 degrees (for medium-rare), 30 to 50 minutes.
5. Transfer roast to carving board, tent with foil, and let rest for 20 minutes. Discard tarragon sprigs. Stir broth into cooking liquid and simmer over medium-high heat until thickened slightly, about 2 minutes. Off heat, stir in minced tarragon and season with pepper to taste; cover to keep warm.
6. Discard twine. Slice roast thin and transfer to serving platter. Spoon sauce over meat and serve.

Nutrition Info:
- 190 cal., 6g fat (1g sag. fat), 80mg chol, 240mg sod., 3g carb (1g sugars, 1g fiber), 28g pro.

Stewed Beef And Ale

Servings: 4 | Cooking Time:1 Hour And 40 Minutes

Ingredients:
- 1 pound boneless top round steak, cut in 1/4 inch × 3 1/2–inch strips
- 1 cup chopped onion
- 1 (14.5-ounce) can stewed tomatoes
- 1 cup beer
- 1 teaspoon sugar (optional)
- 1/4 teaspoon salt
- 1/4 teaspoon black pepper

Directions:
1. Place a large nonstick skillet over medium-high heat until hot. Coat the skillet with nonstick cooking spray. Working in two batches, add half of the beef strips and brown, stirring constantly, and set aside on a separate plate. Repeat with the remaining beef strips.
2. Recoat the skillet with nonstick cooking spray, add the onions, and cook 4 minutes or until the onions are translucent, stirring frequently. Add the remaining ingredients, including the beef and any accumulated juices.
3. Bring to a boil over high heat, then reduce the heat, cover tightly, and simmer 1 hour and 30 minutes or until the beef is very tender. Using the back of a spoon, mash the beef pieces to thicken the dish slightly.

Nutrition Info:
- 180 cal., 3g fat (1g sag. fat), 60mg chol, 390mg sod., 10g carb (7g sugars, 2g fiber), 25g pro.

Grapefruit-zested Pork

Servings: 4 | Cooking Time:6 Minutes

Ingredients:
- 3 tablespoons lite soy sauce
- 1/2–1 teaspoon grapefruit zest
- 3 tablespoons grapefruit juice
- 1 jalapeño pepper, seeded and finely chopped, or 1/8–1/4 teaspoon dried red pepper flakes
- 4 thin lean pork chops with bone in (about 1 1/4 pounds total)

Directions:
1. Combine all ingredients in a large zippered plastic bag. Seal tightly and toss back and forth to coat evenly. Refrigerate overnight or at least 8 hours.
2. Preheat the broiler.
3. Coat the broiler rack and pan with nonstick cooking spray, arrange the pork chops on the rack (discarding the marinade), and broil 2 inches away from the heat source for 3 minutes. Turn and broil 3 minutes longer or until the pork is no longer pink in the center.

Nutrition Info:
- 130 cal., 3g fat (1g sag. fat), 60mg chol, 270mg sod., 2g carb (1g sugars, 0g fiber), 23g pro.

Spicy Tomato Pork Chops

Servings:4 | Cooking Time: 30 Minutes

Ingredients:
- 1 tablespoon olive oil
- 4 boneless pork loin chops (5 ounces each)
- 1 large onion, chopped
- 1 can (8 ounces) tomato sauce
- 1/4 cup water
- 2 teaspoons chili powder
- 1 teaspoon dried oregano
- 1 teaspoon Worcestershire sauce
- 1/2 teaspoon sugar
- 1/2 teaspoon crushed red pepper flakes

Directions:
1. In a large skillet, heat oil over medium heat. Brown pork chops on both sides. Remove; keep warm. In same skillet, cook and stir onion until tender. Stir in remaining ingredients.
2. Return pork to skillet. Bring to a boil. Reduce heat; simmer, covered, 15-20 minutes or until tender. Let stand for 5 minutes before serving. Serve the pork chops with the sauce

Nutrition Info:
- 257 cal., 12g fat (3g sat. fat), 68mg chol., 328mg sod., 8g carb. (3g sugars, 2g fiber), 29g pro.

Soups, Stews, And Chilis Recipes

Chickpea And Kale Soup..36

Creamy Potato Soup With Green Onions...............36

Salmon Dill Soup 37

Shrimp Pad Thai Soup...37

Creamy Curried Cauliflower Soup 38

Pumpkin Turkey Chili 38

Mushroom And Wheat Berry Soup 39

Garlic-chicken And Wild Rice Soup 39

Soups, Stews, And Chilis Recipes

Chickpea And Kale Soup

Servings:8 | Cooking Time: 15 Minutes

Ingredients:
- ¼ cup extra-virgin olive oil
- 2 onions, chopped
- 2 fennel bulbs, stalks discarded, bulbs halved, cored, and chopped
- 4 ounces Spanish-style chorizo sausage, cut into ¼-inch pieces
- Salt and pepper
- 6 garlic cloves, minced
- ¼ teaspoon red pepper flakes
- 8 cups unsalted chicken broth
- 2 (15-ounce) cans no-salt-added chickpeas, rinsed
- 12 ounces kale, stemmed and chopped
- 1 teaspoon sherry vinegar, plus extra for seasoning
- 1 ounce Pecorino Romano cheese, grated (½ cup)
- ¼ cup chopped fresh parsley

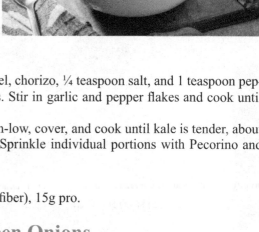

Directions:
1. Heat oil in Dutch oven over medium heat until shimmering. Add onions, fennel, chorizo, ¼ teaspoon salt, and 1 teaspoon pepper and cook until vegetables are softened and lightly browned, 8 to 10 minutes. Stir in garlic and pepper flakes and cook until fragrant, about 30 seconds.
2. Stir in broth, chickpeas, and kale and bring to simmer. Reduce heat to medium-low, cover, and cook until kale is tender, about 15 minutes. Stir in vinegar and season with extra vinegar and pepper to taste. Sprinkle individual portions with Pecorino and parsley before serving.

Nutrition Info:
- 280 cal., 14g fat (3g sag. fat), 15mg chol, 500mg sod., 24g carb (6g sugars, 7g fiber), 15g pro.

Creamy Potato Soup With Green Onions

Servings: 3 | Cooking Time:15 Minutes

Ingredients:
- 2 cups fat-free milk
- 1 pound baking potatoes, peeled and diced
- 3 tablespoons no-trans-fat margarine (35% vegetable oil)
- 1/4 teaspoon salt
- 1/4 teaspoon black pepper
- 3 tablespoons finely chopped green onions, green and white parts

Directions:
1. Bring the milk just to a boil in a large saucepan over high heat (catch it before it comes to a full boil).
2. Add the potatoes and return just to a boil. Reduce the heat, cover tightly, and simmer 12 minutes or until the potatoes are tender.
3. Remove from the heat and add the margarine, salt, and pepper. Using a whisk or potato masher or handheld electric mixer, mash the mixture until thickened, but still lumpy.
4. Spoon into individual bowls and sprinkle each serving with 1 tablespoon onions.

Nutrition Info:
- 200 cal., 5g fat (1g sag. fat), 5mg chol, 360mg sod., 32g carb (9g sugars, 2g fiber), 8g pro.

Salmon Dill Soup

Servings:2 | Cooking Time: 30 Minutes

Ingredients:
- 1 large potato, peeled and cut into 1 1/2-inch pieces
- 1 large carrot, cut into 1/2-inch-thick slices
- 1 1/2 cups water
- 1 cup reduced-sodium chicken broth
- 5 medium fresh mushrooms, halved
- 1 tablespoon all-purpose flour
- 1/4 cup reduced-fat evaporated milk
- 1/4 cup shredded part-skim mozzarella cheese
- 1/2 pound salmon fillet, cut into 1 1/2-inch pieces
- 1/4 teaspoon pepper
- 1/8 teaspoon salt
- 1 tablespoon chopped fresh dill

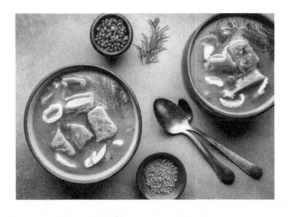

Directions:
1. Place first four ingredients in a saucepan; bring to a boil. Reduce heat to medium; cook, uncovered, until vegetables are tender, 10-15 minutes.
2. Add mushrooms. In a small bowl, mix flour and milk until smooth; stir into soup. Return to a boil; cook and stir until mushrooms are tender. Reduce the heat to medium; stir in the cheese until melted.
3. Reduce heat to medium-low. Add salmon; cook, uncovered, until fish just begins to flake easily with a fork, 3-4 minutes. Stir in pepper and salt. Sprinkle with dill.

Nutrition Info:
- 398 cal., 14g fat (4g sat. fat), 71mg chol., 647mg sod., 37g carb. (7g sugars, 3g fiber), 30g pro.

Shrimp Pad Thai Soup

Servings:8 | Cooking Time: 30 Minutes

Ingredients:
- 1 tablespoon sesame oil
- 2 shallots, thinly sliced
- 1 Thai chili pepper or serrano pepper, seeded and finely chopped
- 1 can (28 ounces) no-salt-added crushed tomatoes
- 1/4 cup creamy peanut butter
- 2 tablespoons reduced-sodium soy sauce or fish sauce
- 6 cups reduced-sodium chicken broth
- 1 pound uncooked shrimp (31-40 per pound), peeled and deveined
- 6 ounces uncooked thick rice noodles
- 1 cup bean sprouts
- 4 green onions, sliced
- Chopped peanuts and additional chopped Thai chili pepper, optional
- Lime wedges

Directions:
1. In a 6-qt. stockpot, heat oil over medium heat. Add shallots and chili pepper; cook and stir 4-6 minutes or until tender. Stir in crushed tomatoes, peanut butter and soy sauce until blended; add broth. Bring to a boil; cook, uncovered, 15 minutes to allow flavors to blend.
2. Add shrimp and noodles; cook 4-6 minutes longer or until shrimp turn pink and noodles are tender. Top each serving with bean sprouts, green onions and, if desired, chopped peanuts and additional chopped chili pepper. Serve with lime wedges.

Nutrition Info:
- 252 cal., 7g fat (1g sat. fat), 69mg chol., 755mg sod., 31g carb. (5g sugars, 4g fiber), 17g pro.

Creamy Curried Cauliflower Soup

Servings:8 | Cooking Time:20 Minutes

Ingredients:
- 1 head cauliflower (2 pounds)
- ¼ cup extra-virgin olive oil
- 1 tablespoon grated fresh ginger
- 1 tablespoon curry powder
- 1 leek, white and light green parts only, halved length-wise, sliced thin, and washed thoroughly
- 1 small onion, halved and sliced thin
- Salt and pepper
- 4½ cups water
- ½ cup canned light coconut milk
- 1 teaspoon lime juice

Directions:
1. Pull off outer leaves of cauliflower and trim stem. Using paring knife, cut around core to remove; slice core thin and reserve. Cut heaping 1 cup of ½-inch florets from head of cauliflower; set aside. Cut remaining cauliflower crosswise into ½-inch-thick slices.

2. Heat 3 tablespoons oil in large saucepan over medium heat until shimmering. Add ginger and curry powder and cook until fragrant, about 1 minute. Add leek, onion, and ¼ teaspoon salt and cook, stirring often, until softened but not browned, about 7 minutes. Stir in water, sliced core, and half of sliced cauliflower. Bring to simmer and cook for 15 minutes. Stir in remaining sliced cauliflower and simmer until cauliflower is tender and crumbles easily, 15 to 20 minutes.

3. Meanwhile, heat remaining 1 tablespoon oil in 8-inch skillet over medium heat until shimmering. Add reserved florets and cook, stirring often, until golden brown, 6 to 8 minutes; transfer to bowl and season with pepper to taste.

4. Working in batches, process soup in blender until smooth, about 1 minute. Return soup to clean saucepan and bring to brief simmer over medium-low heat. Off heat, stir in coconut milk, lime juice, and ½ teaspoon salt. Top individual portions with florets before serving.

Nutrition Info:
- 130 cal., 9g fat (2g sag. fat), 0mg chol, 270mg sod., 11g carb (4g sugars, 3g fiber), 3g pro.

Pumpkin Turkey Chili

Servings:8 | Cooking Time:30 Minutes

Ingredients:
- 1 pound ground turkey
- 1 tablespoon plus 2 cups water, plus extra as needed
- Salt and pepper
- ¼ teaspoon baking soda
- 4 dried ancho chiles, stemmed, seeded, and torn into ½-inch pieces (1 cup)
- 1½ tablespoons ground cumin
- 1½ teaspoons ground coriander
- 1½ teaspoons dried oregano
- 1½ teaspoons paprika
- 1 (28-ounce) can no-salt-added whole peeled tomatoes
- 2 tablespoons extra-virgin olive oil
- 2 onions, chopped fine
- 2 red bell peppers, stemmed, seeded, and cut into ½-inch pieces
- 6 garlic cloves, minced
- 1 cup canned unsweetened pumpkin puree
- 2 (15-ounce) cans no-salt-added black beans, rinsed
- ¼ cup chopped fresh cilantro
- Lime wedges

Directions:
1. Toss turkey, 1 tablespoon water, ¼ teaspoon salt, and baking soda in bowl until thoroughly combined. Set aside for 20 minutes.

2. Toast anchos in Dutch oven over medium-high heat, stirring frequently, until fragrant, 4 to 6 minutes; transfer to food processor and let cool slightly. Add cumin, coriander, oregano, paprika, and 1 teaspoon pepper and process until finely ground, about 2 minutes; transfer to bowl. Process tomatoes and their juice in now-empty food processor until smooth, about 30 seconds.

3. Heat oil in now-empty pot over medium heat until shimmering. Add onions, bell peppers, and ¾ teaspoon salt and cook until softened, 8 to 10 minutes. Increase heat to medium-high, add turkey, and cook, breaking up meat with wooden spoon, until no longer pink, 4 to 6 minutes. Stir in spice mixture and garlic and cook until fragrant, about 30 seconds. Stir in tomatoes, pumpkin, and remaining 2 cups water and bring to simmer. Reduce heat to low, cover, and cook, stirring occasionally, for 1 hour.

4. Stir in beans, cover, and cook until slightly thickened, about 45 minutes. (If chili begins to stick to bottom of pot or looks too thick, stir in extra water as needed.) Season with pepper to taste. Sprinkle individual portions with cilantro and serve with lime wedges.

Nutrition Info:
- 240 cal., 6g fat (1g sag. fat), 20mg chol, 460mg sod., 26g carb (6g sugars, 9g fiber), 22g pro.

Mushroom And Wheat Berry Soup

Servings:8 | Cooking Time:10 Minutes

Ingredients:

- 1 cup wheat berries, rinsed
- 3 tablespoons extra-virgin olive oil
- 1½ pounds cremini mushrooms, trimmed and sliced thin
- ¼ teaspoon salt
- 1 onion, chopped fine
- 6 garlic cloves, minced
- 2 teaspoons no-salt-added tomato paste
- 1 cup dry sherry
- 8 cups unsalted chicken broth
- 1 tablespoon low-sodium soy sauce
- 1 sprig fresh thyme
- 1 bay leaf
- ½ ounce dried shiitake mushrooms, finely ground using spice grinder
- 4 ounces mustard greens, stemmed and chopped
- ¼ teaspoon grated lemon zest plus 2 teaspoons juice

Directions:

1. Toast wheat berries in Dutch oven over medium heat, stirring often, until fragrant and beginning to darken, about 5 minutes; transfer to bowl.

2. Heat 2 tablespoons oil in now-empty pot over medium heat until shimmering. Add cremini mushrooms and salt, cover, and cook until mushrooms have released their liquid, about 3 minutes. Uncover, increase heat to medium-high, and continue to cook, stirring occasionally, until mushrooms are dry and begin to brown, 5 to 7 minutes; transfer to plate.

3. Heat remaining 1 tablespoon oil in now-empty pot over medium heat until shimmering. Add onion and cook until softened, about 5 minutes. Stir in garlic and tomato paste and cook until slightly darkened, about 2 minutes.

4. Stir in sherry, scraping up any browned bits, and cook until nearly evaporated, about 2 minutes. Stir in wheat berries, broth, soy sauce, thyme sprig, bay leaf, and shiitakes and bring to simmer. Reduce heat to low, cover, and cook until wheat berries are tender but still chewy, 45 minutes to 1 hour.

5. Discard thyme sprig and bay leaf. Off heat, stir in cremini mushrooms and any accumulated juices, mustard greens, and lemon zest. Cover and let sit until greens are wilted, about 5 minutes. Stir in lemon juice. Serve.

Nutrition Info:

- 210 cal., 6g fat (1g sag. fat), 0mg chol, 280mg sod., 26g carb (4g sugars, 5g fiber), 10g pro.

Garlic-chicken And Wild Rice Soup

Servings:6 | Cooking Time:50 Minutes

Ingredients:

- 3 tablespoons extra-virgin olive oil
- ½ cup minced garlic (about 25 cloves)
- 2 carrots, peeled and sliced ¼ inch thick
- 1 onion, chopped fine
- 1 celery rib, minced
- Salt and pepper
- 2 teaspoons minced fresh thyme or ½ teaspoon dried
- 1 teaspoon no-salt-added tomato paste
- 6 cups unsalted chicken broth
- 2 bay leaves
- ⅔ cup wild rice, rinsed
- 8 ounces boneless, skinless chicken breasts, trimmed of all visible fat and cut into ¾-inch pieces
- 3 ounces (3 cups) baby spinach
- ¼ cup chopped fresh parsley

Directions:

1. Heat oil and garlic in Dutch oven over medium-low heat, stirring occasionally, until garlic is light golden and fragrant, 3 to 5 minutes. Increase heat to medium and add carrots, onion, celery, and ¼ teaspoon salt. Cook, stirring occasionally, until vegetables are softened and lightly browned, 10 to 12 minutes.

2. Stir in thyme and tomato paste and cook until fragrant, about 30 seconds. Stir in broth and bay leaves, scraping up any browned bits. Stir in rice and bring to simmer. Reduce heat to medium-low, cover, and cook until rice is tender, 40 to 50 minutes.

3. Discard bay leaves. Reduce heat to low and stir in chicken and spinach. Cook, stirring occasionally, until chicken is cooked through and spinach is wilted, 3 to 5 minutes. Off heat, stir in parsley and season with pepper to taste. Serve.

Nutrition Info:

- 240 cal., 9g fat (1g sag. fat), 30mg chol, 280mg sod., 25g carb (3g sugars, 4g fiber), 17g pro.

Special Treats Recipes

Pineapple Breeze Torte 41

Banana-pineapple Cream Pies 41

No-fuss Banana Ice Cream 42

Chocolate-dipped Strawberry Meringue Roses 42

Warm Figs With Goat Cheese And Honey 43

Saucy Spiced Pears 43

Pomegranate And Nut Chocolate Clusters 43

Peaches, Blackberries, And Strawberries With Basil And Pepper 44

Apple Cinnamon Rollups 44

Special Treats Recipes

Pineapple Breeze Torte

Servings:12 | Cooking Time: 5 Minutes

Ingredients:
- 3 packages (3 ounces each) soft ladyfingers, split
- FILLING
- 1 package (8 ounces) fat-free cream cheese
- 3 ounces cream cheese, softened
- 1/3 cup sugar
- 2 teaspoons vanilla extract
- 1 carton (8 ounces) frozen reduced-fat whipped topping, thawed
- TOPPING
- 1/3 cup sugar
- 3 tablespoons cornstarch
- 1 can (20 ounces) unsweetened crushed pineapple, undrained

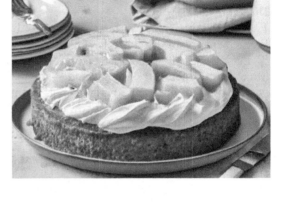

Directions:
1. Line bottom and sides of an ungreased 9-in. springform pan with ladyfinger halves; reserve remaining ladyfingers for layering.
2. Beat cream cheeses, sugar and vanilla until smooth; fold in whipped topping. Spread half of the mixture over bottom ladyfingers. Layer with the remaining ladyfingers, overlapping as needed. Spread with the remaining filling. Refrigerate, covered, while preparing topping.
3. In a small saucepan, mix sugar and cornstarch; stir in pineapple. Bring to a boil over medium heat, stirring constantly; cook and stir until thickened, 1-2 minutes. Cool the mixture completely.
4. Spread topping gently over torte. Refrigerate, covered, until set, at least 4 hours. Remove rim from pan.

Nutrition Info:
- 243 cal., 7g fat (5g sat. fat), 87mg chol., 156mg sod., 39g carb. (27g sugars, 1g fiber), 6g pro.

Banana-pineapple Cream Pies

Servings:2 | Cooking Time: 15 Minutes

Ingredients:
- 1/4 cup cornstarch
- 1/4 cup sugar
- 1 can (20 ounces) unsweetened crushed pineapple, undrained
- 3 medium bananas, sliced
- Two 9-inch graham cracker crusts (about 6 ounces each)
- 1 carton (8 ounces) frozen whipped topping, thawed

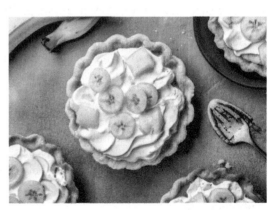

Directions:
1. In a large saucepan, combine cornstarch and sugar. Stir in pineapple until blended. Bring to a boil; cook and stir 1-2 minutes or until thickened.
2. Arrange bananas over bottom of each crust; spread the pineapple mixture over tops. Refrigerate at least 1 hour before serving. Top with the whipped topping.

Nutrition Info:
- 205 cal., 8g fat (3g sat. fat), 0 chol., 122mg sod., 33g carb. (23g sugars, 1g fiber), 1g pro.

No-fuss Banana Ice Cream

Servings:1 | Cooking Time: 15 Minutes

Ingredients:
- 6 very ripe bananas
- ½ cup heavy cream
- 1 tablespoon vanilla extract
- 1 teaspoon lemon juice
- ¼ teaspoon salt
- ¼ teaspoon ground cinnamon

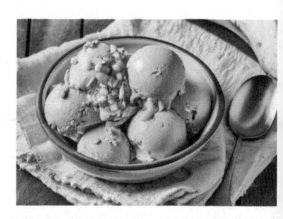

Directions:

1. Peel bananas, place in large zipper-lock bag, and press out excess air. Freeze bananas until solid, at least 8 hours.

2. Let bananas sit at room temperature to soften slightly, about 15 minutes. Slice into ½-inch-thick rounds and place in food processor. Add cream, vanilla, lemon juice, salt, and cinnamon and process until smooth, about 5 minutes, scraping down sides of bowl as needed.

3. Transfer mixture to airtight container and freeze until firm, at least 2 hours or up to 5 days. Serve.

Nutrition Info:
- 160 cal., 6g fat (3g sag. fat), 15mg chol, 75mg sod., 28g carb (18g sugars, 3g fiber), 1g pro.

Chocolate-dipped Strawberry Meringue Roses

Servings:3 | Cooking Time: 40 Minutes

Ingredients:
- 3 large egg whites
- 1/4 cup sugar
- 1/4 cup freeze-dried strawberries
- 1 package (3 ounces) strawberry gelatin
- 1/2 teaspoon vanilla extract, optional
- 1 cup 60% cacao bittersweet chocolate baking chips, melted

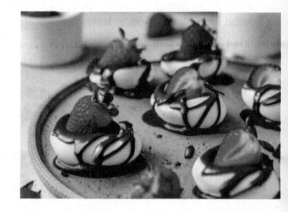

Directions:

1. Place egg whites in a large bowl; let stand at room temperature 30 minutes. Preheat oven to 225°.

2. Place sugar and strawberries in a food processor; process until powdery. Add gelatin; pulse to blend.

3. Beat egg whites on medium speed until foamy, adding vanilla if desired. Gradually add gelatin mixture, 1 tablespoon at a time, beating on high after each addition until sugar is dissolved. Continue beating until stiff glossy peaks form.

4. Cut a small hole in the tip of a pastry bag or in a corner of a food-safe plastic bag; insert a #1M star tip. Transfer meringue to bag. Pipe 2-in. roses 1 1/2 in. apart onto parchment paper-lined baking sheets.

5. Bake 40-45 minutes or until set and dry. Turn off oven (do not open oven door); leave meringues in oven 1 1/2 hours. Remove from oven; cool completely on baking sheets.

6. Remove meringues from paper. Dip bottoms in melted chocolate; allow excess to drip off. Place on waxed paper; let stand until set, about 45 minutes. Store in an airtight container at room temperature.

Nutrition Info:
- 33 cal., 1g fat (1g sat. fat), 0 chol., 9mg sod., 6g carb. (5g sugars, 0 fiber), 1g pro.

Warm Figs With Goat Cheese And Honey

Servings:6 | Cooking Time:4 Minutes

Ingredients:
- 2 ounces goat cheese
- 9 fresh figs, halved lengthwise
- 18 walnut halves, toasted
- 2 tablespoons honey

Directions:
1. Adjust oven rack to middle position and heat oven to 500 degrees. Spoon heaping ½ teaspoon goat cheese onto each fig half and arrange on parchment paper–lined rimmed baking sheet. Bake figs until heated through, about 4 minutes; transfer to serving platter.
2. Place 1 walnut half on top of each fig half and drizzle with honey. Serve.

Nutrition Info:
- 140 cal., 6g fat (2g sag. fat), 5mg chol, 45mg sod., 21g carb (18g sugars, 3g fiber), 3g pro.

Saucy Spiced Pears

Servings:4 | Cooking Time: 20 Minutes

Ingredients:
- 1/2 cup orange juice
- 2 tablespoons butter
- 2 tablespoons sugar
- 2 teaspoons lemon juice
- 1 teaspoon vanilla extract
- 1 teaspoon ground ginger
- 1/4 teaspoon ground cinnamon
- 1/8 teaspoon salt
- 1/8 teaspoon ground allspice
- 1/8 teaspoon cayenne pepper, optional
- 3 large Bosc pears (about 1 3/4 pounds), cored, peeled and sliced
- Thinly sliced fresh mint leaves, optional

Directions:
1. In a large skillet, combine the first nine ingredients and, if desired, cayenne. Cook over medium-high heat 1-2 minutes or until butter is melted, stirring occasionally.
2. Add pears; bring to a boil. Reduce heat to medium; cook, uncovered, 3-4 minutes or until sauce is slightly thickened and pears are crisp-tender, stirring occasionally. Cool slightly. If desired, top with mint.

Nutrition Info:
- 192 cal., 6g fat (4g sat. fat), 15mg chol., 130mg sod., 36g carb. (26g sugars, 5g fiber), 1g pro.

Pomegranate And Nut Chocolate Clusters

Servings:12 | Cooking Time: 30 Minutes

Ingredients:
- ⅓ cup pecans, toasted and chopped
- ¼ cup shelled pistachios, toasted and chopped
- 2 tablespoons unsweetened flaked coconut, toasted
- 2 tablespoons pomegranate seeds
- 3 ounces semisweet chocolate, chopped fine

Directions:
1. Line rimmed baking sheet with parchment paper. Combine pecans, pistachios, coconut, and pomegranate seeds in bowl.
2. Microwave 2 ounces chocolate in bowl at 50 percent power, stirring often, until about two-thirds melted, 45 to 60 seconds. Remove bowl from microwave; stir in remaining 1 ounce chocolate until melted. If necessary, microwave chocolate at 50 percent power for 5 seconds at a time until melted.
3. Working quickly, measure 1 teaspoon melted chocolate onto prepared sheet and spread into 2½-inch wide circle using back of spoon. Repeat with remaining chocolate, spacing circles 1½ inches apart.
4. Sprinkle pecan mixture evenly over chocolate and press gently to adhere. Refrigerate until chocolate is firm, about 30 minutes. Serve.

Nutrition Info:
- 80 cal., 6g fat (2g sag. fat), 0mg chol, 0mg sod., 6g carb (5g sugars, 1g fiber), 1g pro.

Peaches, Blackberries, And Strawberries With Basil And Pepper

Servings:6 | Cooking Time:15 Minutes

Ingredients:
- Nectarines can be substituted for the peaches.
- 2 teaspoons sugar
- 2 tablespoons chopped fresh basil
- ½ teaspoon pepper
- 3 peaches, halved, pitted, and cut into ½-inch pieces
- 10 ounces (2 cups) blackberries
- 10 ounces strawberries, hulled and quartered (2 cups)
- 1 tablespoon lime juice, plus extra for seasoning

Directions:
1. Combine sugar, basil, and pepper in large bowl. Using rubber spatula, press mixture into side of bowl until sugar becomes damp, about 30 seconds. Add peaches, blackberries, and strawberries and gently toss to combine. Let sit at room temperature, stirring occasionally, until fruit releases its juices, 15 to 30 minutes. Stir in lime juice and season with extra lime juice to taste. Serve.

Nutrition Info:
- 70 cal., 0g fat (0g sag. fat), 0mg chol, 0mg sod., 18g carb (13g sugars, 5g fiber), 2g pro.

Apple Cinnamon Rollups

Servings:6 | Cooking Time:26 Minutes

Ingredients:
- 2 apples (6 ounces each), cored, halved, and sliced thin
- 1 tablespoon unsalted butter, melted and cooled
- 2 teaspoons lemon juice
- 1 teaspoon ground cinnamon
- ½ teaspoon ground ginger
- ¼ teaspoon salt
- 2 tablespoons sugar
- 1 (9½ by 9-inch) sheet puff pastry, thawed
- 2 tablespoons apricot preserves

Directions:
1. Adjust oven rack to middle position and heat oven to 375 degrees. Toss apples with melted butter, lemon juice, ½ teaspoon cinnamon, ginger, and salt in bowl. Spread apples in single layer on parchment paper–lined rimmed baking sheet and bake until softened, about 10 minutes. Set aside until cool enough to handle, about 10 minutes.
2. Line clean baking sheet with parchment and lightly spray with canola oil spray. Combine sugar and remaining ½ teaspoon cinnamon in bowl.
3. Roll pastry into 12 by 10-inch rectangle on lightly floured counter, with long side parallel to counter edge. Brush preserves evenly over top and sprinkle with cinnamon sugar. Using sharp knife or pizza wheel, cut pastry lengthwise into six 10 by 2-inch strips.
4. Working with 1 strip of dough at a time, shingle 12 apple slices, peel side out, along length of dough, leaving 1-inch border of dough on one side. Fold bare inch of dough over bottom of apple slices, leaving top of apple slices exposed. Roll up dough and apples into tight pinwheel and place, apple side up, on prepared sheet.
5. Bake until golden brown and crisp, 22 to 26 minutes, rotating sheet halfway through baking. Let Danish cool on sheet for 15 minutes before serving.

Nutrition Info:
- 240 cal., 12g fat (6g sag. fat), 5mg chol, 240mg sod., 36g carb (13g sugars, 2g fiber), 3g pro.

Poultry Recipes

Caribbean Delight...46

Asian Lettuce Wraps..46

Oven-fried Chicken Drumsticks...........................47

Grilled Chicken Kebabs With Tomato-feta Salad 47

Chicken Enchiladas 48

Turkey Sausage Zucchini Boats 48

Turkey Cutlets With Barley And Broccoli 49

Cumin-crusted Chicken Thighs With Cauliflower Couscous49

Poultry Recipes

Caribbean Delight

Servings:6 | Cooking Time: 10 Minutes

Ingredients:
- 2 tablespoons finely chopped onion
- 1/4 cup butter, cubed
- 2 garlic cloves, minced
- 1/3 cup white vinegar
- 1/3 cup lime juice
- 1/4 cup sugar
- 2 tablespoons curry powder
- 1 teaspoon salt
- 1/4 to 1/2 teaspoon cayenne pepper
- 6 boneless skinless chicken breast halves (4 ounces each)

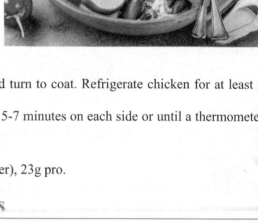

Directions:
1. In a small saucepan, saute onion in butter until tender. Add garlic; cook 1 minute longer. Stir in the vinegar, lime juice, sugar, curry, salt and cayenne. Place chicken in a large resealable plastic bag; add onion mixture. Seal bag and turn to coat. Refrigerate chicken for at least 2 hours.
2. Drain and discard marinade. Grill chicken, uncovered, over medium heat for 5-7 minutes on each side or until a thermometer reads 170°.

Nutrition Info:
- 162 cal., 5g fat (2g sat. fat), 70mg chol., 224mg sod., 4g carb. (3g sugars, 0 fiber), 23g pro.

Asian Lettuce Wraps

Servings:4 | Cooking Time: 25 Minutes

Ingredients:
- 1 tablespoon canola oil
- 1 pound lean ground turkey
- 1 jalapeno pepper, seeded and minced
- 2 green onions, thinly sliced
- 2 garlic cloves, minced
- 2 tablespoons minced fresh basil
- 2 tablespoons lime juice
- 2 tablespoons reduced-sodium soy sauce
- 1 to 2 tablespoons chili garlic sauce
- 1 tablespoon sugar or sugar substitute blend equivalent to 1 tablespoon sugar
- 12 Bibb or Boston lettuce leaves
- 1 medium cucumber, julienned
- 1 medium carrot, julienned
- 2 cups bean sprouts

Directions:
1. In a skillet, heat oil over medium heat. Add turkey; cook 6-8 minutes or until no longer pink, breaking into crumbles. Add jalapeno, green onions and garlic; cook 2 minute longer. Stir in basil, lime juice, soy sauce, chili garlic sauce and sugar; heat through.
2. To serve, place turkey mixture in lettuce leaves; top with cucumber, carrot and bean sprouts. Fold lettuce over filling.

Nutrition Info:
- 259 cal., 12g fat (3g sat. fat), 78mg chol., 503mg sod., 12g carb. (6g sugars, 3g fiber), 26g pro.

Oven-fried Chicken Drumsticks

Servings:4 | Cooking Time: 40 Minutes

Ingredients:
- 1 cup fat-free plain Greek yogurt
- 1 tablespoon Dijon mustard
- 2 garlic cloves, minced
- 8 chicken drumsticks (4 ounces each), skin removed
- 1/2 cup whole wheat flour
- 1 1/2 teaspoons paprika
- 1 teaspoon baking powder
- 1 teaspoon salt
- 1 teaspoon pepper
- Olive oil-flavored cooking spray

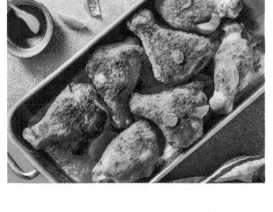

Directions:
1. In a large resealable plastic bag, combine yogurt, mustard and garlic. Add chicken; seal bag and turn to coat. Refrigerate 8 hours or overnight.
2. Preheat oven to 425°. In another plastic bag, mix flour, paprika, baking powder, salt and pepper. Remove the chicken from marinade and add, one piece at a time, to flour mixture; close bag and shake to coat. Place on a wire rack over a baking sheet; spritz with cooking spray. Bake 40-45 minutes or until a thermometer reads 180°.

Nutrition Info:
- 227 cal., 7g fat (1g sat. fat), 81mg chol., 498mg sod., 9g carb. (2g sugars, 1g fiber), 31g pro.

Grilled Chicken Kebabs With Tomato-feta Salad

Servings:4 | Cooking Time:25 Minutes

Ingredients:
- ¼ cup extra-virgin olive oil
- 1 teaspoon grated lemon zest plus 3 tablespoons juice
- 3 garlic cloves, minced
- 1 tablespoon minced fresh oregano
- Salt and pepper
- 1 pound cherry tomatoes, halved
- 3 ounces feta cheese, crumbled (¾ cup)
- ¼ cup thinly sliced red onion
- ¼ cup plain low-fat yogurt
- 1½ pounds boneless, skinless chicken breasts, trimmed of all visible fat and cut into 1-inch pieces

Directions:
1. Whisk oil, lemon zest and juice, garlic, oregano, ¼ teaspoon salt, and ½ teaspoon pepper together in medium bowl. Reserve half of oil mixture in separate medium bowl. Add tomatoes, feta, and onion to remaining oil mixture and toss to coat. Season with pepper to taste and set salad aside for serving.
2. Whisk yogurt into reserved oil mixture. Set aside half of yogurt dressing for serving. Add chicken to remaining yogurt dressing and toss to coat. Thread chicken onto four 12-inch metal skewers.
3. FOR A CHARCOAL GRILL Open bottom vent completely. Light large chimney starter filled with charcoal briquettes (6 quarts). When top coals are partially covered with ash, pour evenly over grill. Set cooking grate in place, cover, and open lid vent completely. Heat grill until hot, about 5 minutes.
4. FOR A GAS GRILL Turn all burners to high, cover, and heat grill until hot, about 15 minutes. Leave all burners on high.
5. Place skewers on grill and cook, turning occasionally, until chicken is well browned and registers 160 degrees, about 10 minutes. Using tongs, slide chicken off skewers onto serving platter. Serve chicken with salad and reserved dressing.

Nutrition Info:
- 400 cal., 21g fat (6g sag. fat), 145mg chol, 410mg sod., 9g carb (6g sugars, 2g fiber), 43g pro.

Chicken Enchiladas

Servings:6 | Cooking Time:25 Minutes

Ingredients:
- 1 tablespoon canola oil
- 1 onion, chopped fine
- ½ teaspoon salt
- 3 garlic cloves, minced
- 1 tablespoon chipotle chile powder
- 2 teaspoons ground cumin
- 1 (15-ounce) can no-salt-added tomato sauce
- 1¼ cups water
- 1 pound boneless, skinless chicken breasts, trimmed of all visible fat
- 4 ounces cheddar cheese, shredded (1 cup)
- 1 (4-ounce) can chopped green chiles, drained and chopped fine
- ½ cup minced fresh cilantro, plus ¼ cup leaves
- 12 (6-inch) corn tortillas
- Canola oil spray
- ¾ cup low-fat sour cream
- Lime wedges

Directions:

1. Adjust oven rack to middle position and heat oven to 350 degrees. Heat oil in large saucepan over medium heat until shimmering. Add onion and salt and cook until softened, 5 to 7 minutes. Stir in garlic, chile powder, and cumin and cook until fragrant, about 30 seconds. Stir in tomato sauce and water, bring to simmer, and cook until slightly thickened, about 5 minutes. Add chicken and bring to simmer. Reduce heat to medium-low, cover, and cook until chicken registers 160 degrees, 10 to 15 minutes.

2. Transfer chicken to cutting board, let cool slightly, then shred into bite-size pieces using 2 forks. Strain sauce through fine-mesh strainer into bowl, pressing on solids to extract as much liquid as possible. Transfer solids to large bowl and stir in chicken, ½ cup strained sauce, ½ cup cheddar, chiles, and minced cilantro.

3. Wrap tortillas in clean dish towel and microwave until pliable, 30 to 90 seconds. Top each tortilla with ⅓ cup chicken mixture, roll tightly, and lay seam side down in 13 by 9-inch baking dish (2 columns of 6 tortillas will fit neatly across width of dish).

4. Lightly spray tops of enchiladas with oil spray. Pour remaining sauce over enchiladas and sprinkle remaining ½ cup cheddar evenly over top. Cover dish with aluminum foil and bake until enchiladas are hot throughout, about 25 minutes. Remove foil and continue to bake until cheese browns slightly, about 5 minutes.

5. Let enchiladas rest for 5 minutes. Sprinkle with cilantro leaves and serve with sour cream and lime wedges.

Nutrition Info:
- 360 cal., 15g fat (5g sag. fat), 80mg chol, 480mg sod., 32g carb (6g sugars, 6g fiber), 28g pro.

Turkey Sausage Zucchini Boats

Servings:6 | Cooking Time: 35 Minutes

Ingredients:
- 6 medium zucchini
- 1 pound lean ground turkey
- 1 small onion, chopped
- 1 celery rib, chopped
- 1 garlic clove, minced
- 1 1/2 teaspoons Italian seasoning
- 3/4 teaspoon salt
- 1/4 teaspoon cayenne pepper
- 1/4 teaspoon paprika
- 1 cup salad croutons, coarsely crushed
- 1 cup shredded part-skim mozzarella cheese, divided

Directions:

1. Preheat oven to 350°. Cut each zucchini lengthwise in half. Scoop out pulp, leaving a 1/4-in. shell; chop pulp.

2. In a large skillet, cook turkey, onion, celery, garlic and seasonings over medium heat 6-8 minutes or until turkey is no longer pink, breaking up turkey into crumbles. Stir in croutons, 1/2 cup cheese and zucchini pulp. Spoon into zucchini shells.

3. Transfer to two ungreased 13x9-in. baking dishes; add 1/4 in. water. Bake, covered, 30-35 minutes or until zucchini is tender. Sprinkle with the remaining cheese. Bake, uncovered, for about 5 minutes or until cheese is melted.

Nutrition Info:
- 240 cal., 11g fat (4g sat. fat), 63mg chol., 556mg sod., 13g carb. (5g sugars, 2g fiber), 23g pro.

Turkey Cutlets With Barley And Broccoli

Servings:4 | Cooking Time:22 Minutes.

Ingredients:

- ¼ cup extra-virgin olive oil
- 1 onion, chopped fine
- 1 cup pearled barley, rinsed
- 3 garlic cloves, minced
- 2 cups unsalted chicken broth
- ¼ cup minced fresh parsley
- Salt and pepper
- 4 (4-ounce) turkey cutlets, ¼ inch thick, trimmed of all visible fat
- 1 lemon, zested to yield ½ teaspoon, halved and seeded
- 1 pound broccoli florets, cut into 1-inch pieces
- ⅛ teaspoon red pepper flakes
- 2 tablespoons grated Parmesan cheese

Directions:

1. Heat 1 tablespoon oil in large saucepan over medium heat until shimmering. Add onion and cook until softened, about 5 minutes. Stir in barley and garlic and cook, stirring often, until lightly golden and fragrant, about 3 minutes.

2. Stir in broth and bring to simmer. Reduce heat to low, cover, and cook until barley is tender and broth is absorbed, 20 to 40 minutes. Add parsley, 1 tablespoon oil, and ⅛ teaspoon salt and gently fluff with fork to combine; cover to keep warm.

3. Meanwhile, pat cutlets dry with paper towels and sprinkle with ¼ teaspoon salt and ⅛ teaspoon pepper. Heat 1 teaspoon oil in 12-inch nonstick skillet over medium-high heat until shimmering. Cook lemon halves cut side down until browned, about 2 minutes; set aside. Heat 2 teaspoons oil in now-empty skillet until shimmering. Cook cutlets until well browned and tender, about 2 minutes per side. Transfer to plate and tent with aluminum foil.

4. Heat remaining 1 tablespoon oil in now-empty skillet over medium-high heat until just smoking. Add broccoli and cook, without stirring, until beginning to brown, about 2 minutes. Add 3 tablespoons water, cover, and cook until broccoli is bright green but still crisp, about 2 minutes. Uncover and continue to cook until water has evaporated and broccoli is crisp-tender, about 2 minutes. Off heat, add lemon zest, pepper flakes, ⅛ teaspoon salt, and ⅛ teaspoon pepper and toss to combine. Squeeze lemon halves over barley and cutlets. Serve with broccoli, sprinkling individual portions with Parmesan.

Nutrition Info:

- 500 cal., 17g fat (2g sag. fat), 45mg chol, 480mg sod., 49g carb (4g sugars, 12g fiber), 40g pro.

Cumin-crusted Chicken Thighs With Cauliflower Couscous

Servings:4 | Cooking Time:25 Minutes

Ingredients:

- 8 (3-ounce) boneless, skinless chicken thighs, trimmed of all visible fat
- 2 teaspoons cumin seeds
- Salt and pepper
- 2 tablespoons canola oil
- 1 head cauliflower (2 pounds), cored and cut into ½-inch pieces
- 1 teaspoon paprika
- ½ cup pomegranate seeds
- ½ cup chopped fresh mint
- 1½ teaspoons grated lime zest, plus lime wedges for serving

Directions:

1. Pat chicken thighs dry with paper towels and sprinkle with 1 teaspoon cumin seeds, ¼ teaspoon salt, and ¼ teaspoon pepper. Heat 1 tablespoon oil in 12-inch nonstick skillet over medium-high heat until just smoking. Cook thighs, turning as needed, until well browned and register 175 degrees, about 8 minutes. Transfer chicken to plate, tent with aluminum foil, and let rest while preparing cauliflower.

2. Working in 2 batches, pulse cauliflower in food processor to ¼- to ⅛-inch pieces, about 6 pulses. Heat remaining 1 tablespoon oil in now-empty skillet over medium-high heat until shimmering. Add cauliflower, paprika, ⅛ teaspoon salt, ¼ teaspoon pepper, and remaining 1 teaspoon cumin seeds and cook, stirring occasionally, until just tender, about 7 minutes. Off heat, stir in pomegranate seeds, chopped mint, and lime zest. Serve chicken with couscous and lime wedges.

Nutrition Info:

- 320 cal., 15g fat (2g sag. fat), 160mg chol, 410mg sod., 10g carb (5g sugars, 4g fiber), 36g pro.

Slow Cooker Favorites Recipes

Slow Cooker Mushroom Chicken & Peas...........................51

Spiced Pork Tenderloin With Carrots And Radishes...........51

Teriyaki Beef Stew 52

Italian Cabbage Soup...52

Sweet Onion & Red Bell Pepper Topping.....................53

Beets With Oranges And Walnuts..............................53

Butternut Squash With Whole Grains 53

Pork Loin With Fennel, Oranges, And Olives 54

Turkey Chili..54

Slow Cooker Favorites Recipes

Slow Cooker Mushroom Chicken & Peas

Servings:4 | Cooking Time: 3 Hours 10 Minutes

Ingredients:
- 4 boneless skinless chicken breast halves (6 ounces each)
- 1 envelope onion mushroom soup mix
- 1 cup water
- 1/2 pound sliced baby portobello mushrooms
- 1 medium onion, chopped
- 4 garlic cloves, minced
- 2 cups frozen peas, thawed

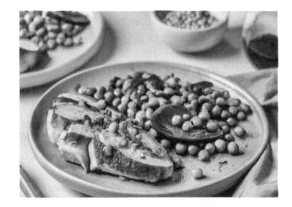

Directions:
1. Place chicken in a 3-qt. slow cooker. Sprinkle with soup mix, pressing to help seasonings adhere to chicken. Add water, mushrooms, onion and garlic.
2. Cook, covered, on low 3-4 hours or until chicken is tender (a thermometer inserted in chicken should read at least 165°). Stir in peas; cook, covered, 10 minutes longer or until heated through.

Nutrition Info:
- 292 cal., 5g fat (1g sat. fat), 94mg chol., 566mg sod., 20g carb. (7g sugars, 5g fiber), 41g pro.

Spiced Pork Tenderloin With Carrots And Radishes

Servings:4 | Cooking Time: 2 Hours

Ingredients:
- 1½ pounds carrots, peeled and sliced ¼ inch thick on bias
- 10 radishes, trimmed and sliced ¼ inch thick
- ¼ cup unsalted chicken broth
- 3 tablespoons extra-virgin olive oil
- 1 teaspoon ground cumin
- 1 teaspoon paprika
- 1 (1-pound) pork tenderloin, trimmed of all visible fat
- Salt and pepper
- 2 tablespoons lime juice
- 2 tablespoons minced fresh cilantro
- 1 teaspoon minced canned chipotle chile in adobo sauce

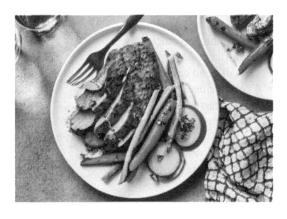

Directions:
1. Microwave carrots and ¼ cup water in covered bowl, stirring occasionally, until crisp-tender, about 8 minutes. Drain carrots and transfer to oval slow cooker. Stir in radishes and broth.
2. Microwave 1 teaspoon oil, cumin, and paprika in bowl until fragrant, about 30 seconds; let cool slightly. Rub tenderloin with spice mixture and sprinkle with ¼ teaspoon salt and ⅛ teaspoon pepper. Nestle tenderloin into slow cooker, cover, and cook until pork registers 145 degrees, 1 to 2 hours on low.
3. Transfer tenderloin to carving board, tent with aluminum foil, and let rest for 5 minutes.
4. Whisk remaining 8 teaspoons oil, lime juice, cilantro, and chipotle together in bowl, then season dressing with pepper to taste. Drain vegetables from cooker and transfer to large bowl. Stir in 2 tablespoons of dressing and season with pepper to taste. Slice tenderloin ½ inch thick and serve with vegetables and remaining dressing.

Nutrition Info:

- 300 cal., 14g fat (2g sag. fat), 75mg chol, 350mg sod., 20g carb (9g sugars, 6g fiber), 26g pro.

Teriyaki Beef Stew

Servings:8 | Cooking Time: 6 1/2 Hours

Ingredients:
- 2 pounds beef stew meat
- 1 bottle (12 ounces) ginger beer or ginger ale
- 1/4 cup teriyaki sauce
- 2 garlic cloves, minced
- 2 tablespoons sesame seeds
- 2 tablespoons cornstarch
- 2 tablespoons cold water
- 2 cups frozen peas, thawed
- Hot cooked rice, optional

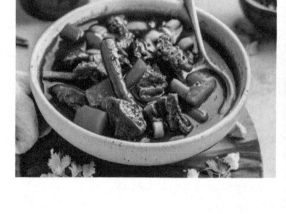

Directions:
1. In a nonstick skillet, brown beef in batches. Transfer to a 3-qt. slow cooker.
2. In a small bowl, combine the ginger beer, teriyaki sauce, garlic and sesame seeds; pour over beef. Cover and cook on low for 6-8 hours or until the meat is tender.
3. Combine cornstarch and cold water until smooth; gradually stir into stew. Stir in peas. Cover and cook on high for 30 minutes or until thickened. Serve with rice if desired.

Nutrition Info:
- 310 cal., 12g fat (4g sat. fat), 94mg chol., 528mg sod., 17g carb. (9g sugars, 2g fiber), 33g pro.

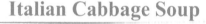

Italian Cabbage Soup

Servings:8 | Cooking Time: 6 Hours

Ingredients:
- 4 cups chicken stock
- 1 can (6 ounces) tomato paste
- 1 small head cabbage (about 1 1/2 pounds), shredded
- 4 celery ribs, chopped
- 2 large carrots, chopped
- 1 small onion, chopped
- 1 can (15 1/2 ounces) great northern beans, rinsed and drained
- 2 garlic cloves, minced
- 2 fresh thyme sprigs
- 1 bay leaf
- 1/2 teaspoon salt
- Shredded Parmesan cheese, optional

Directions:
1. In a 5- or 6-qt. slow cooker, whisk together stock and tomato paste. Stir in the vegetables, beans, garlic and seasonings. Cook, covered, on low until vegetables are tender, 6-8 hours.
2. Remove thyme sprigs and bay leaf. If desired, serve with cheese.

Nutrition Info:
- 111 cal., 0 fat (0 sat. fat), 0 chol., 537mg sod., 21g carb. (7g sugars, 6g fiber), 8g pro.

Sweet Onion & Red Bell Pepper Topping

Servings:4 | Cooking Time: 4 Hours

Ingredients:
- 4 large sweet onions, thinly sliced (about 8 cups)
- 4 large sweet red peppers, thinly sliced (about 6 cups)
- 1/2 cup cider vinegar
- 1/4 cup packed brown sugar
- 2 tablespoons canola oil
- 2 tablespoons honey
- 2 teaspoons celery seed
- 3/4 teaspoon crushed red pepper flakes
- 1/2 teaspoon salt

Directions:
1. In a 5- or 6-qt. slow cooker, combine all ingredients. Cook, covered, on low 4-5 hours or until the vegetables are tender. Serve with a slotted spoon.

Nutrition Info:
- 76 cal., 2g fat (0 sat. fat), 0 chol., 84mg sod., 14g carb. (11g sugars, 2g fiber), 1g pro.

Beets With Oranges And Walnuts

Servings:4 | Cooking Time:7hours

Ingredients:
- 1½ pounds beets, trimmed
- 2 oranges
- ¼ cup white wine vinegar
- 1½ tablespoons extra-virgin olive oil
- Salt and pepper
- ¼ cup walnuts, toasted and chopped coarse
- 2 tablespoons minced fresh chives

Directions:
1. Wrap beets individually in aluminum foil and place in oval slow cooker. Add ½ cup water, cover, and cook until beets are tender, 6 to 7 hours on low or 4 to 5 hours on high.
2. Transfer beets to cutting board and carefully remove foil (watch for steam). When beets are cool enough to handle, rub off skins with paper towels and cut into ½-inch-thick wedges.
3. Cut away peel and pith from oranges. Quarter oranges and slice crosswise into ½-inch-thick pieces. Whisk vinegar, oil, ¼ teaspoon salt, and ¼ teaspoon pepper together in large bowl. Add beets and orange pieces and toss to coat. Season with pepper to taste. Sprinkle with walnuts and chives and serve.

Nutrition Info:
- 190 cal., 10g fat (1g sag. fat), 0mg chol, 260mg sod., 25g carb (18g sugars, 7g fiber), 4g pro.

Butternut Squash With Whole Grains

Servings:12 | Cooking Time: 4 Hours

Ingredients:
- 1 medium butternut squash (about 3 pounds), cut into 1/2-inch cubes
- 1 cup uncooked whole grain brown and red rice blend
- 1 medium onion, chopped
- 1/2 cup water
- 3 garlic cloves, minced
- 2 teaspoons minced fresh thyme or 1/2 teaspoon dried thyme
- 1/2 teaspoon salt
- 1/4 teaspoon pepper
- 1 can (14 1/2 ounces) vegetable broth
- 1 package (6 ounces) fresh baby spinach

Directions:
1. In a 4-qt. slow cooker, combine the first eight ingredients. Stir in broth.
2. Cook, covered, on low 4-5 hours or until grains are tender. Stir in spinach before serving.

Nutrition Info:
- 97 cal., 1g fat (0 sat. fat), 0 chol., 252mg sod., 22g carb. (3g sugars, 4g fiber), 3g pro.

Pork Loin With Fennel, Oranges, And Olives

Servings:8 | Cooking Time: 2 Hours

Ingredients:
- 1 (2-pound) boneless center-cut pork loin roast, fat trimmed to ⅛ inch
- 1 teaspoon herbes de Provence
- Salt and pepper
- 1 tablespoon extra-virgin olive oil
- 3 fennel bulbs, stalks discarded, bulbs halved, cored, and sliced thin
- ½ cup dry white wine
- 2 garlic cloves, minced
- 4 oranges, plus 1 tablespoon grated orange zest
- ½ cup pitted kalamata olives, chopped
- 2 tablespoons minced fresh tarragon

Directions:
1. Pat roast dry with paper towels and sprinkle with herbes de Provence, ½ teaspoon salt, and ¼ teaspoon pepper. Heat oil in 12-inch skillet over medium-high heat until just smoking. Brown roast on all sides, 7 to 10 minutes; transfer to plate.
2. Add fennel and wine to now-empty skillet, cover, and cook, stirring occasionally, until fennel begins to soften, about 5 minutes. Uncover and continue to cook until fennel is dry and lightly browned, about 5 minutes. Stir in garlic and cook until fragrant, about 30 seconds; transfer to oval slow cooker. Nestle roast fat side up into slow cooker. Cover and cook until pork registers 140 degrees, 1 to 2 hours on low.
3. Transfer roast to carving board, tent with aluminum foil, and let rest for 15 minutes. Meanwhile, cut away peel and pith from oranges. Quarter oranges, then slice crosswise into ½-inch-thick pieces. Stir orange segments, orange zest, olives, and ¼ teaspoon salt into fennel mixture and let sit until heated through, about 5 minutes. Stir in tarragon and season with pepper to taste. Slice pork ½ inch thick and serve with fennel-orange mixture.

Nutrition Info:
- 240 cal., 7g fat (1g sag. fat), 70mg chol., ___ng sod., 15g carb (10g sugars, 4g fiber), 27g pro.

Turkey Chili

Servings:8 | Cooking Time:4hours

Ingredients:
- 2 pounds ground turkey
- 2 tablespoons water
- Salt and pepper
- ½ teaspoon baking soda
- ¼ cup canola oil
- 3 onions, chopped fine
- 1 red bell pepper, stemmed, seeded, and chopped
- ¼ cup no-salt-added tomato paste
- 3 tablespoons chili powder
- 6 garlic cloves, minced
- 1 tablespoon ground cumin
- ¾ teaspoon dried oregano
- 1¼ cups unsalted chicken broth, plus extra as needed
- 2 tablespoons low-sodium soy sauce
- 2 (15-ounce) cans no-salt-added kidney beans, rinsed
- 1 (28-ounce) can no-salt-added diced tomatoes, drained
- 1 (15-ounce) can no-salt-added tomato sauce
- 2 teaspoons minced canned chipotle chile in adobo sauce
- ¼ cup chopped fresh cilantro
- Lime wedges

Directions:
1. Toss turkey with water, ¼ teaspoon salt, and baking soda in bowl until thoroughly combined. Set aside for 20 minutes.
2. Heat oil in 12-inch skillet over medium heat until shimmering. Add onions and bell pepper and cook until softened and lightly browned, 8 to 10 minutes. Stir in tomato paste, chili powder, garlic, cumin, and oregano and cook until fragrant, about 1 minute.
3. Add half of turkey mixture and cook, breaking up turkey with wooden spoon, until no longer pink, about 5 minutes. Repeat with remaining turkey mixture. Stir in broth and soy sauce, scraping up any browned bits; transfer to slow cooker.
4. Stir beans, tomatoes, tomato sauce, and chipotle into slow cooker. Cover and cook until turkey is tender, 4 to 5 hours on low. Break up any remaining large pieces of turkey with spoon. Adjust consistency with extra hot broth as needed. Season with pepper to taste. Sprinkle individual portions with cilantro and serve with lime wedges.

Nutrition Info:
- 320 cal., 9g fat (2g sag. fat), 45mg chol, 500mg sod., 25g carb (8g sugars, 10g fiber), 36g pro.

Potatoes, Pasta, And Whole Grains Recipes

Fusilli With Skillet-roasted Cauliflower, Garlic, And Walnuts 56

Taco-spiced Rice...56

Creamy Parmesan Polenta...57

Spaghetti With Spinach, Beans, Tomatoes, And Garlic Chips 57

Warm Farro With Mushrooms And Thyme.........................58

Fusilli With Zucchini, Tomatoes, And Pine Nuts 58

Spaghetti And Meatballs...59

Warm Farro With Fennel And Parmesan...........................59

Potatoes, Pasta, And Whole Grains Recipes

Fusilli With Skillet-roasted Cauliflower, Garlic, And Walnuts

Servings:6 | Cooking Time:20 Minutes

Ingredients:
- ¼ cup extra-virgin olive oil
- 1 head cauliflower (2 pounds), cored and cut into ½-inch florets
- Salt and pepper
- 3 garlic cloves, minced
- 1 teaspoon grated lemon zest plus 1–2 tablespoons juice
- ¼ teaspoon red pepper flakes
- 12 ounces (4½ cups) 100 percent whole-wheat fusilli
- 1 ounce Parmesan cheese, grated (½ cup)
- 2 tablespoons chopped fresh parsley
- ¼ cup walnuts, toasted and chopped coarse

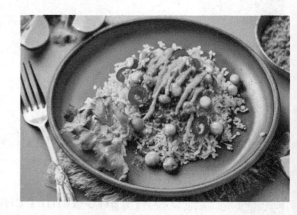

Directions:
1. Combine 2 tablespoons oil and cauliflower florets in 12-inch nonstick skillet and sprinkle with ½ teaspoon salt and ¼ teaspoon pepper. Cover skillet and cook over medium-high heat until florets start to brown and edges just start to become translucent (do not lift lid), about 5 minutes. Remove lid and continue to cook, stirring every 2 minutes, until florets turn golden brown in many spots, about 12 minutes.
2. Push cauliflower to sides of skillet. Add 1 tablespoon oil, garlic, lemon zest, and pepper flakes to center and cook, stirring with rubber spatula, until fragrant, about 30 seconds. Stir garlic mixture into cauliflower and continue to cook, stirring occasionally, until cauliflower is tender but still firm, about 3 minutes.
3. Meanwhile, bring 4 quarts water to boil in large pot. Add pasta and 1 teaspoon salt and cook, stirring often, until al dente. Reserve 1 cup cooking water, then drain pasta and return it to pot.
4. Add cauliflower mixture, ¼ cup Parmesan, parsley, ½ cup reserved cooking water, 1 tablespoon lemon juice, and remaining 1 tablespoon oil to pasta and toss to combine. Season with extra lemon juice to taste and adjust consistency with reserved cooking water as needed. Sprinkle individual portions with walnuts and remaining ¼ cup Parmesan. Serve.

Nutrition Info:
- 360 cal., 16g fat (2g sag. fat), 5mg chol, 390mg sod., 44g carb (4g sugars, 10g fiber), 13g pro.

Taco-spiced Rice

Servings: 4 | Cooking Time:11 Minutes

Ingredients:
- 1 1/4 cups water (divided use)
- 1/2 cup instant brown rice
- 1 medium red bell pepper, chopped
- 1 medium onion, chopped
- 1 tablespoon taco seasoning (available in packets)
- 1 tablespoon no-trans-fat margarine (35% vegetable oil), optional

Directions:
1. Bring 1 cup water and the rice to boil in a small saucepan, then reduce the heat, cover tightly, and simmer 10 minutes.
2. Meanwhile, place a large nonstick skillet over medium-high heat until hot. Coat the skillet with nonstick cooking spray and add the peppers and onions. Coat the vegetables with nonstick cooking spray and cook 5 minutes or until the vegetables are tender-crisp.
3. In a small bowl, dissolve the taco seasoning in 1/4 cup water. Stir into the rice, add the margarine, if desired, and stir until well blended.

Nutrition Info:
- 130 cal., 2g fat (0g sag. fat), 0mg chol, 200mg sod., 25g carb (4g sugars, 3g fiber), 3g pro.

Creamy Parmesan Polenta

Servings:6 | Cooking Time: 25 Minutes

Ingredients:
- 5 cups water
- Salt and pepper
- Pinch baking soda
- 1 cup coarse-ground cornmeal
- 1 ounce Parmesan cheese, grated (½ cup)
- ¼ cup minced fresh parsley or basil
- 1 tablespoons extra-virgin olive oil

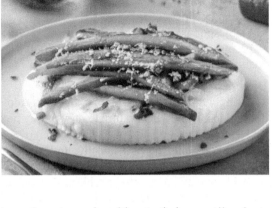

Directions:

1. Bring water to boil in large saucepan over medium-high heat. Stir in ½ teaspoon salt and baking soda. While whisking constantly, slowly pour cornmeal into water in steady stream. Bring mixture to boil, stirring constantly, then reduce heat to lowest setting and cover.

2. After 5 minutes, whisk polenta to smooth out any lumps that may have formed. (Make sure to scrape down sides and bottom of saucepan.) Cover and continue to cook, without stirring, until polenta grains are tender but slightly al dente, about 25 minutes. (Polenta should be loose and barely hold its shape; it will continue to thicken as it cools.)

3. Off heat, stir in Parmesan, parsley, and oil and season with pepper to taste. Cover and let sit for 5 minutes. Serve.

Nutrition Info:
- 100 cal., 4g fat (1g sag. fat), 5mg chol, 300mg sod., 14g carb (0g sugars, 2g fiber), 4g pro.

Spaghetti With Spinach, Beans, Tomatoes, And Garlic Chips

Servings:6 | Cooking Time:18 Minutes

Ingredients:
- 3 tablespoons extra-virgin olive oil
- 8 garlic cloves, peeled (5 sliced thin lengthwise, 3 minced)
- 1 onion, chopped fine
- ¼–½ teaspoon red pepper flakes
- 1¼ pounds curly spinach, stemmed and cut into 1-inch pieces
- ¾ cup unsalted chicken broth
- 1 (14.5-ounce) can no-salt-added diced tomatoes, drained
- Salt and pepper
- 1 (15-ounce) can no-salt-added cannellini beans, rinsed
- ¾ cup pitted kalamata olives, chopped coarse
- 12 ounces 100 percent whole-wheat spaghetti
- 1 ounce Parmesan cheese, grated (½ cup)

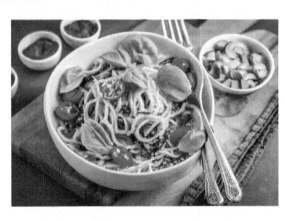

Directions:

1. Cook oil and sliced garlic in 12-inch straight-sided sauté pan over medium heat, stirring often, until garlic turns golden but not brown, about 3 minutes. Using slotted spoon, transfer garlic to paper towel–lined plate; set aside.

2. Add onion to oil left in pan and cook over medium heat until softened and lightly browned, 5 to 7 minutes. Stir in minced garlic and pepper flakes and cook until fragrant, about 30 seconds. Add half of spinach and cook, tossing occasionally, until starting to wilt, about 2 minutes. Add remaining spinach, broth, tomatoes, and ⅛ teaspoon salt and bring to simmer. Reduce heat to medium, cover (pan will be very full), and cook, tossing occasionally, until spinach is completely wilted, about 10 minutes (mixture will be somewhat soupy). Off heat, stir in beans and olives.

3. Meanwhile, bring 4 quarts water to boil in large pot. Add pasta and 1 teaspoon salt and cook, stirring often, until just shy of al dente. Reserve ½ cup cooking water, then drain pasta and return it to pot. Add spinach mixture and cook over medium heat, tossing to combine, until pasta absorbs most of liquid, about 2 minutes.

4. Off heat, stir in Parmesan. Season with pepper to taste and adjust consistency with reserved cooking water as needed. Sprinkle individual portions with garlic chips. Serve.

Nutrition Info:
- 360 cal., 11g fat (1g sag. fat), 5mg chol, 360mg sod., 50g carb (3g sugars, 11g fiber), 15g pro.

Warm Farro With Mushrooms And Thyme

Servings:6 | Cooking Time: 30 Minutes

Ingredients:
- 1½ cups whole farro
- Salt and pepper
- 3 tablespoons extra-virgin olive oil
- 12 ounces cremini mushrooms, trimmed and chopped coarse
- 1 shallot, minced
- 1½ teaspoons minced fresh thyme or ½ teaspoon dried
- 3 tablespoons dry sherry
- 3 tablespoons minced fresh parsley
- 1½ teaspoons sherry vinegar, plus extra for seasoning

Directions:
1. Bring 4 quarts water to boil in large pot. Add farro and 1 teaspoon salt and cook until grains are tender with slight chew, 15 to 30 minutes. Drain farro, return to now-empty pot, and cover to keep warm.
2. Heat 2 tablespoons oil in 12-inch skillet over medium heat until shimmering. Add mushrooms, shallot, thyme, and ¼ teaspoon salt and cook, stirring occasionally, until moisture has evaporated and vegetables start to brown, 8 to 10 minutes. Stir in sherry, scraping up any browned bits, and cook until skillet is almost dry.
3. Add farro and remaining 1 tablespoon oil and cook until heated through, about 2 minutes. Off heat, stir in parsley and vinegar. Season with pepper and extra vinegar to taste and serve.

Nutrition Info:
- 250 cal., 9g fat (1g sag. fat), 0mg chol, 135mg sod., 39g carb (4g sugars, 4g fiber), 7g pro.

Fusilli With Zucchini, Tomatoes, And Pine Nuts

Servings:6 | Cooking Time:30 Minutes

Ingredients:
- 2 pounds zucchini and/or summer squash, halved lengthwise and sliced ½ inch thick
- Kosher salt and pepper
- 3 tablespoons extra-virgin olive oil
- 3 garlic cloves, minced
- ⅛–½ teaspoon red pepper flakes
- 12 ounces (4½ cups) 100 percent whole-wheat fusilli
- 12 ounces grape tomatoes, halved
- ½ cup chopped fresh basil
- 2 tablespoons balsamic vinegar
- ¼ cup grated Parmesan cheese
- ¼ cup pine nuts, toasted

Directions:
1. Toss squash with 1 tablespoon salt in colander and let drain for 30 minutes. Pat squash dry with paper towels and carefully wipe away any residual salt.
2. Heat ½ tablespoon oil in 12-inch nonstick skillet over high heat until just smoking. Add half of squash and cook, turning once, until golden brown and slightly charred, 5 to 7 minutes, reducing heat if squash begins to scorch; transfer to large plate. Repeat with ½ tablespoon oil and remaining squash; transfer to plate.
3. Heat 1 tablespoon oil in now-empty skillet over medium heat until shimmering. Add garlic and pepper flakes and cook until fragrant, about 30 seconds. Stir in squash and cook until heated through, about 30 seconds.
4. Meanwhile, bring 4 quarts water to boil in large pot. Add pasta and 2 teaspoons salt and cook, stirring often, until al dente. Reserve ½ cup cooking water, then drain pasta and return it to pot. Add squash mixture, tomatoes, basil, vinegar, and remaining 1 tablespoon oil and toss to combine. Adjust consistency with reserved cooking water as needed. Sprinkle individual portions with Parmesan and pine nuts.

Nutrition Info:
- 340 cal., 14g fat (2g sag. fat), 5mg chol, 220mg sod., 44g carb (7g sugars, 8g fiber), 12g pro.

Spaghetti And Meatballs

Servings:6 | Cooking Time:40minutes

Ingredients:

- MEATBALLS
- 1 (1¼-ounce) slice 100 percent whole-wheat sandwich bread, crusts removed, torn into pieces
- 1½ tablespoons 1 percent low-fat milk
- ¼ cup grated Parmesan cheese
- 3 tablespoons chopped fresh basil
- 1 large egg yolk
- 2 garlic cloves, minced
- Salt and pepper
- 1½ pounds ground turkey
- 1 tablespoon extra-virgin olive oil

- PASTA AND SAUCE
- 1 onion, chopped fine
- Salt
- 4 garlic cloves, minced
- ½ teaspoon minced fresh oregano
- ⅛ teaspoon red pepper flakes
- 1 (28-ounce) can no-salt-added crushed tomatoes
- 1 (14.5-ounce) can no-salt-added diced tomatoes
- 12 ounces 100 percent whole-wheat spaghetti
- 3 tablespoons shredded fresh basil

Directions:

1. FOR THE MEATBALLS Mash bread and milk together in bowl to smooth paste. Stir in Parmesan, basil, egg yolk, garlic, ½ teaspoon salt, and ¼ teaspoon pepper. Add turkey and combine with hands until mixture is uniformly smooth. Gently form mixture into 1½-inch round meatballs (18 meatballs) and place on large plate. Refrigerate until firm, about 1 hour.

2. Heat oil in 12-inch nonstick skillet over medium heat until just smoking. Brown meatballs on all sides, about 10 minutes. Transfer meatballs to paper towel–lined plate, leaving fat in skillet.

3. FOR THE PASTA AND SAUCE Add onion and ¼ teaspoon salt to fat left in skillet and cook over medium heat until browned, about 8 minutes. Stir in garlic, oregano, and red pepper flakes and cook until fragrant, about 30 seconds. Stir in crushed tomatoes and diced tomatoes with their juices. Bring to simmer, reduce heat to medium-low, and cook until sauce has thickened slightly, about 20 minutes.

4. Add meatballs to sauce and bring to simmer. Cover and cook, turning meatballs occasionally, until cooked through, about 10 minutes.

5. Meanwhile, bring 4 quarts water to boil in large pot. Add pasta and 1 teaspoon salt and cook, stirring often, until al dente. Reserve ½ cup cooking water, then drain pasta and return it to pot.

6. Add basil and several large spoonfuls of sauce (without meatballs) to the pasta and toss to combine. Adjust consistency with reserved cooking water as needed. Divide pasta between six individual bowls. Top each bowl with 3 meatballs and additional sauce. Serve.

Nutrition Info:

- 430 cal., 7g fat (3g sag. fat), 80mg chol, 490mg sod., 49g carb (9g sugars, 10g fiber), 40g pro.

Warm Farro With Fennel And Parmesan

Servings:6 | Cooking Time:30 Minutes

Ingredients:

- 1½ cups whole farro
- Salt and pepper
- 3 tablespoons extra-virgin olive oil
- 1 onion, chopped fine
- 1 small fennel bulb, stalks discarded, bulb halved, cored, and chopped fine

- 3 garlic cloves, minced
- 1 teaspoon minced fresh thyme or ¼ teaspoon dried
- 1 ounce Parmesan cheese, grated (½ cup)
- ¼ cup minced fresh parsley
- 2 teaspoons sherry vinegar, plus extra for seasoning

Directions:

1. Bring 4 quarts water to boil in large pot. Add farro and 1 teaspoon salt and cook until grains are tender with slight chew, 15 to 30 minutes. Drain farro, return to now-empty pot, and cover to keep warm.

2. Heat 2 tablespoons oil in 12-inch skillet over medium heat until shimmering. Add onion, fennel, and ¼ teaspoon salt and cook until softened, 6 to 8 minutes. Stir in garlic and thyme and cook until fragrant, about 30 seconds. Add farro and remaining 1 tablespoon oil and cook until heated through, about 2 minutes. Off heat, stir in Parmesan, parsley, and vinegar. Season with pepper and extra vinegar to taste. Serve.

Nutrition Info:

- 280 cal., 10g fat (1g sag. fat), 5mg chol, 240mg sod., 41g carb (4g sugars, 6g fiber), 9g pro.

Fish & Seafood Recipes

Mustard Vinaigrette With Lemon And Parsley.....................61

Crispy Fish & Chips 61

Creamy Dill Sauce...62

Two-sauce Cajun Fish 62

Lemon-herb Cod Fillets With Garlic Potatoes 63

Asian Snapper With Capers...63

Oven-roasted Salmon 63

Shrimp Avocado Salad...64

Crunchy Tuna Wraps 64

Fish & Seafood Recipes

Mustard Vinaigrette With Lemon And Parsley

Servings:1 | Cooking Time:10 Minutes

Ingredients:
- 3 tablespoons extra-virgin olive oil
- 2 tablespoons lemon juice
- 5 teaspoons whole-grain mustard
- 1 small shallot, minced
- 1 tablespoon water
- 2 teaspoons minced fresh parsley
- Pepper

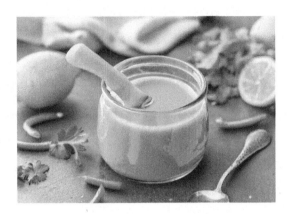

Directions:
1. Whisk oil, lemon juice, mustard, shallot, water, and parsley together in bowl and season with pepper to taste. Let sit for 10 minutes. (Vinaigrette can be refrigerated for up to 24 hours; whisk to recombine before serving.)

Nutrition Info:
- 110 cal., 11g fat (1g sag. fat), 0mg chol, 125mg sod., 1g carb (0g sugars, 0g fiber), 0g pro.

Crispy Fish & Chips

Servings:4 | Cooking Time: 30 Minutes

Ingredients:
- 4 cups frozen steak fries
- 4 salmon fillets (6 ounces each)
- 1 to 2 tablespoons prepared horseradish
- 1 tablespoon grated Parmesan cheese
- 1 tablespoon Worcestershire sauce
- 1 teaspoon Dijon mustard
- 1/4 teaspoon salt
- 1/2 cup panko (Japanese) bread crumbs
- Cooking spray

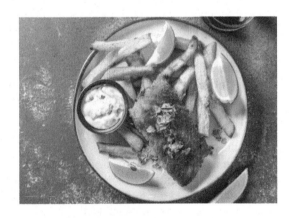

Directions:
1. Preheat oven to 450°. Arrange steak fries in a single layer on a baking sheet. Bake on lowest oven rack 18-20 minutes or until light golden brown.
2. Meanwhile, place salmon on a foil-lined baking sheet coated with cooking spray. In a small bowl, mix horseradish, cheese, Worcestershire sauce, mustard and salt; stir in panko. Press mixture onto fillets. Spritz tops with cooking spray.
3. Bake salmon on middle oven rack 8-10 minutes or until fish just begins to flake easily with a fork. Serve with fries.

Nutrition Info:
- 419 cal., 20g fat (4g sat. fat), 86mg chol., 695mg sod., 26g carb. (2g sugars, 2g fiber), 32g pro.

Creamy Dill Sauce

Servings:1 | Cooking Time:30 Minutes

Ingredients:
- This creamy sauce goes especially well with salmon.
- ¼ cup mayonnaise
- 2 tablespoons low-fat sour cream
- 1 small shallot, minced
- 1 tablespoon lemon juice
- 1 tablespoon minced fresh dill
- Water
- Pepper

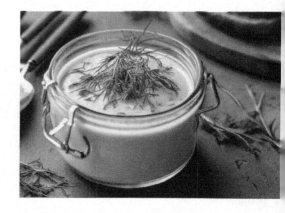

Directions:
1. Combine mayonnaise, sour cream, shallot, lemon juice, and dill in bowl. Add water as needed to thin sauce consistency and season with pepper to taste. Cover and refrigerate for 30 minutes before serving. (Sauce can be refrigerated for up to 24 hours.)

Nutrition Info:
- 100 cal., 11g fat (2g sag. fat), 5mg chol, 95mg sod., 1g carb (1g sugars, 0g fiber), 1g pro.

Two-sauce Cajun Fish

Servings: 4 | Cooking Time:12–15 Minutes

Ingredients:
- 4 (4-ounce) tilapia filets (or any mild, lean white fish filets), rinsed and patted dry
- 1/2 teaspoon seafood seasoning
- 1 (14.5-ounce) can stewed tomatoes with Cajun seasonings, well drained
- 2 tablespoons no-trans-fat margarine (35% vegetable oil)

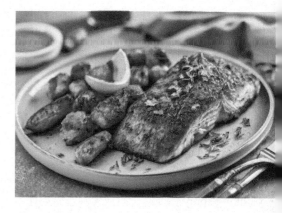

Directions:
1. Preheat the oven to 400°F.
2. Coat a broiler rack and pan with nonstick cooking spray, arrange the fish filets on the rack about 2 inches apart, and sprinkle them evenly with the seafood seasoning.
3. Place the tomatoes in a blender and puree until just smooth. Set aside 1/4 cup of the mixture in a small glass bowl.
4. Spoon the remaining tomatoes evenly over the top of each filet and bake 12–15 minutes or until the filets are opaque in the center.
5. Meanwhile, add the margarine to the reserved 1/4 cup tomato mixture and microwave on HIGH 20 seconds or until the mixture is just melted. Stir to blend well.
6. Place the filets on a serving platter, spoon the tomato-margarine mixture over the center of each filet, and sprinkle each lightly with chopped fresh parsley, if desired.

Nutrition Info:
- 150 cal., 5g fat (1g sag. fat), 50mg chol, 250mg sod., 4g carb (3g sugars, 1g fiber), 23g pro.

Lemon-herb Cod Fillets With Garlic Potatoes

Servings:4 | Cooking Time:40 Minutes

Ingredients:

- 1½ pounds russet potatoes, unpeeled, sliced into ¼-inch-thick rounds
- ¼ cup extra-virgin olive oil
- 3 garlic cloves, minced
- Salt and pepper
- 4 (6-ounce) skinless cod fillets, 1 to 1½ inches thick
- 4 sprigs fresh thyme
- 1 lemon, sliced into ¼-inch-thick rounds

Directions:

1. Adjust oven rack to lower-middle position and heat oven to 425 degrees. Toss potatoes, 2 tablespoons oil, garlic, ⅛ teaspoon salt, and ¼ teaspoon pepper together in bowl. Microwave, uncovered, until potatoes are just tender, 12 to 14 minutes, stirring halfway through microwaving.

2. Transfer potatoes to 13 by 9-inch baking dish and press gently into even layer. Pat cod dry with paper towels, rub with remaining 2 tablespoons oil, and sprinkle with ¼ teaspoon salt and ⅛ teaspoon pepper. Arrange skinned side down on top of potatoes, then place thyme sprigs and lemon slices on top. Bake until cod flakes apart when gently prodded with paring knife and registers 140 degrees, 15 to 18 minutes. Slide spatula underneath potatoes and cod and carefully transfer to individual serving plates. Serve.

Nutrition Info:

- 400 cal., 15g fat (2g sag. fat), 75mg chol, 280mg sod., 32g carb (1g sugars, 2g fiber), 34g pro.

Asian Snapper With Capers

Servings:4 | Cooking Time: 20 Minutes

Ingredients:

- 4 red snapper fillets (6 ounces each)
- 4 1/2 teaspoons Mongolian Fire oil or sesame oil
- 1/4 cup apple jelly
- 3 tablespoons ketchup
- 2 tablespoons capers, drained
- 1 tablespoon lemon juice
- 1 tablespoon reduced-sodium soy sauce
- 1 teaspoon grated fresh gingerroot

Directions:

1. In a large skillet, cook the fillets in oil over medium heat for 3-5 minutes on each side or until fish flakes easily with a fork; remove and keep warm.

2. Stir the jelly, ketchup, capers, lemon juice, soy sauce and ginger into skillet. Cook and stir for 2-3 minutes or until slightly thickened; serve alongside the red snapper.

Nutrition Info:

- 275 cal., 7g fat (1g sat. fat), 60mg chol., 494mg sod., 17g carb. (15g sugars, 0 fiber), 34g pro.

Oven-roasted Salmon

Servings:4 | Cooking Time:10 Minutes

Ingredients:

- 1 (1½-pound) skin-on salmon fillet, 1 inch thick
- 1 teaspoon extra-virgin olive oil
- ¼ teaspoon salt
- ⅛ teaspoon pepper

Directions:

1. Adjust oven rack to lowest position, place aluminum foil–lined rimmed baking sheet on rack, and heat oven to 500 degrees. Cut salmon crosswise into 4 fillets, then make 4 or 5 shallow slashes about an inch apart along skin side of each piece, being careful not to cut into flesh. Pat fillets dry with paper towels, rub with oil, and sprinkle with salt and pepper.

2. Once oven reaches 500 degrees, reduce oven temperature to 275 degrees. Remove sheet from oven and carefully place salmon, skin-side down, on hot sheet. Roast until centers are still translucent when checked with tip of paring knife and register 125 degrees (for medium-rare), 4 to 6 minutes.

3. Slide spatula along underside of fillets and transfer to individual serving plates or serving platter, leaving skin behind; discard skin. Serve.

Nutrition Info:

- 360 cal., 24g fat (5g sag. fat), 95mg chol, 250mg sod., 0g carb (0g sugars, 0g fiber), 35g pro.

Shrimp Avocado Salad

Servings:6 | Cooking Time: 25 Minutes

Ingredients:
- 1 pound peeled and deveined cooked shrimp, coarsely chopped
- 2 plum tomatoes, seeded and chopped
- 2 green onions, chopped
- 1/4 cup finely chopped red onion
- 1 jalapeno pepper, seeded and minced
- 1 serrano pepper, seeded and minced
- 2 tablespoons minced fresh cilantro
- 2 tablespoons lime juice
- 2 tablespoons seasoned rice vinegar
- 2 tablespoons olive oil
- 1 teaspoon adobo seasoning
- 3 medium ripe avocados, peeled and cubed
- Bibb lettuce leaves
- Lime wedges

Directions:
1.Place first seven ingredients in a large bowl. Mix lime juice, vinegar, oil and adobo seasoning; stir into shrimp mixture. Refrigerate, covered, to allow flavors to blend, about 1 hour.
2.To serve, stir in avocados. Serve over lettuce. Serve with lime wedges.

Nutrition Info:
- 252 cal., 16g fat (2g sat. fat), 115mg chol., 523mg sod., 11g carb. (3g sugars, 5g fiber), 17g pro.

Crunchy Tuna Wraps

Servings:2 | Cooking Time: 10 Minutes

Ingredients:
- 1 pouch (6.4 ounces) light tuna in water
- 1/4 cup finely chopped celery
- 1/4 cup chopped green onions
- 1/4 cup sliced water chestnuts, chopped
- 3 tablespoons chopped sweet red pepper
- 2 tablespoons reduced-fat mayonnaise
- 2 teaspoons prepared mustard
- 2 spinach tortillas (8 inches), room temperature
- 1 cup shredded lettuce

Directions:
1.In a small bowl, mix the first seven ingredients until blended. Spread over tortillas; sprinkle with lettuce. Roll up tightly jelly-roll style.

Nutrition Info:
- 312 cal., 10g fat (2g sat. fat), 38mg chol., 628mg sod., 34g carb. (2g sugars, 3g fiber), 23g pro.

Vegetables, Fruit And Side Dishes Recipes

Herbed Potato Packet 66

Fresh Lemon Roasted Brussels Sprouts 66

Sautéed Swiss Chard With Garlic...67

Crunchy Pear And Cilantro Relish 67

Spaghetti Squash With Garlic And Parmesan 68

Balsamic Zucchini Saute 68

Roasted Asparagus...68

Tomato-onion Green Beans..69

Roasted Beets 69

Broiled Eggplant With Basil...69

Vegetables, Fruit And Side Dishes Recipes

Herbed Potato Packet

Servings:4 | Cooking Time: 25 Minutes

Ingredients:
- 1 pound baby red potatoes (about 16), halved
- 1/4 cup cranberry juice
- 2 tablespoons butter, cubed
- 1 teaspoon each minced fresh dill, oregano, rosemary and thyme
- 1/2 teaspoon salt
- 1/8 teaspoon pepper

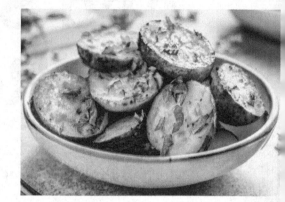

Directions:
1. In a large bowl, combine all the ingredients; place on a piece of heavy-duty foil (about 18x12-in. rectangle). Fold foil around mixture, sealing tightly.
2. Grill, covered, over medium heat 25-30 minutes or until potatoes are tender. Open foil carefully to allow steam to escape.

Nutrition Info:
- 117 cal., 6g fat (4g sat. fat), 15mg chol., 351mg sod., 15g carb. (3g sugars, 1g fiber), 2g pro.

Fresh Lemon Roasted Brussels Sprouts

Servings: 4 | Cooking Time:20 Minutes

Ingredients:
- 1 pound fresh Brussels sprouts, ends trimmed and halved
- 2 tablespoons extra-virgin olive oil, divided
- Juice and zest of 1 medium lemon
- 2 teaspoons Worcestershire sauce
- 1/4 teaspoon pepper

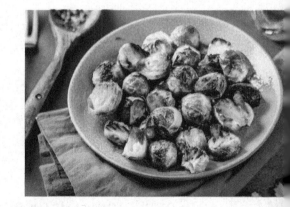

Directions:
1. Preheat oven 425°F.
2. Toss Brussels sprouts with 1 tablespoon oil, place in a single layer on a foil-lined baking sheet. Roast 10 minutes, stir, and cook 10 minutes or until just tender and beginning to brown.
3. Remove, toss with remaining ingredients and 1/4 teaspoon salt, if desired.

Nutrition Info:
- 115 cal., 7g fat (1g sag. fat), 0mg chol, 55mg sod., 13g carb (3g sugars, 5g fiber), 4g pro.

Sautéed Swiss Chard With Garlic

Servings:6 | Cooking Time:8 Minutes

Ingredients:
- 2 tablespoons extra-virgin olive oil
- 3 garlic cloves, sliced thin
- 1½ pounds Swiss chard, stems sliced ¼ inch thick on bias, leaves sliced into ½-inch-wide strips
- 2 teaspoons lemon juice
- Pepper

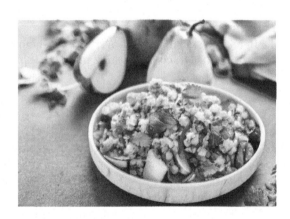

Directions:

1. Heat oil in 12-inch nonstick skillet over medium-high heat until just shimmering. Add garlic and cook, stirring constantly, until lightly browned, 30 to 60 seconds. Add chard stems and cook, stirring occasionally, until spotty brown and crisp-tender, about 6 minutes.

2. Add two-thirds of chard leaves and cook, tossing with tongs, until just starting to wilt, 30 to 60 seconds. Add remaining chard leaves and continue to cook, stirring frequently, until leaves are tender, about 3 minutes. Off heat, stir in lemon juice and season with pepper to taste. Serve.

Nutrition Info:
- 60 cal., 5g fat (0g sag. fat), 0mg chol, 220mg sod., 5g carb (1g sugars, 2g fiber), 2g pro.

Crunchy Pear And Cilantro Relish

Servings: 4 | Cooking Time: 6 Minutes

Ingredients:
- 2 firm medium pears, peeled, cored, and finely chopped (about 1/4-inch cubes)
- 3/4 teaspoon lime zest
- 3 tablespoons lime juice
- 1 1/4 tablespoons sugar
- 3 tablespoons chopped cilantro or mint

Directions:

1. Place all ingredients in a bowl and toss well.
2. Serve immediately for peak flavor and texture.

Nutrition Info:
- 50 cal., 0g fat (0g sag. fat), 0mg chol, 0mg sod., 14g carb (9g sugars, 3g fiber), 0g pro.

Spaghetti Squash With Garlic And Parmesan

Servings:6 | Cooking Time:30 Minutes

Ingredients:
- 1 spaghetti squash (2½ pounds), halved lengthwise and seeded
- 2 tablespoons extra-virgin olive oil
- Salt and pepper
- ¼ cup grated Parmesan cheese
- 1 tablespoon chopped fresh basil
- 1 teaspoon lemon juice
- 1 garlic clove, minced

Directions:
1. Adjust oven rack to middle position and heat oven to 450 degrees. Brush cut sides of squash with 1 tablespoon oil and sprinkle with ½ teaspoon salt and ¼ teaspoon pepper. Lay squash cut side down in 13 by 9-inch baking dish. Roast squash until just tender and tip of paring knife can be slipped into flesh with slight resistance, 25 to 30 minutes.
2. Flip squash over and let cool slightly. Holding squash with clean dish towel over large bowl, use fork to scrape squash flesh from skin while shredding it into fine pieces.
3. Drain excess liquid from bowl, then gently stir Parmesan, basil, lemon juice, garlic, and remaining 1 tablespoon oil into squash. Season with pepper to taste and serve.

Nutrition Info:
- 100 cal., 6g fat (1g sag. fat), 0mg chol, 260mg sod., 10g carb (4g sugars, 2g fiber), 2g pro.

Balsamic Zucchini Saute

Servings:4 | Cooking Time: 20 Minutes

Ingredients:
- 1 tablespoon olive oil
- 3 medium zucchini, cut into thin slices
- 1/2 cup chopped sweet onion
- 1/2 teaspoon salt
- 1/2 teaspoon dried rosemary, crushed
- 1/4 teaspoon pepper
- 2 tablespoons balsamic vinegar
- 1/3 cup crumbled feta cheese

Directions:
1. In a large skillet, heat oil over medium-high heat; saute zucchini and onion until crisp-tender, 6-8 minutes. Stir in the seasonings. Add vinegar; cook and stir 2 minutes. Top with cheese.

Nutrition Info:
- 94 cal., 5g fat (2g sat. fat), 5mg chol., 398mg sod., 9g carb. (6g sugars, 2g fiber), 4g pro.

Roasted Asparagus

Servings:6 | Cooking Time:10 Minutes

Ingredients:
- 2 pounds thick asparagus, trimmed
- 2 tablespoons plus 2 teaspoons extra-virgin olive oil
- ½ teaspoon salt
- ¼ teaspoon pepper

Directions:
1. Adjust oven rack to lowest position, place rimmed baking sheet on rack, and heat oven to 500 degrees. Peel bottom halves of asparagus spears until white flesh is exposed, then toss with 2 tablespoons oil, salt, and pepper.
2. Transfer asparagus to preheated sheet and spread into single layer. Roast, without moving asparagus, until undersides of spears are browned, tops are bright green, and tip of paring knife inserted at base of largest spear meets little resistance, 8 to 10 minutes. Transfer asparagus to serving platter and drizzle with remaining 2 teaspoons oil. Serve.

Nutrition Info:
- 80 cal., 6g fat (1g sag. fat), 0mg chol, 190mg sod., 4g carb (2g sugars, 2g fiber), 3g pro.

Tomato-onion Green Beans

Servings:6 | Cooking Time: 30 Minutes

Ingredients:
- 2 tablespoons olive oil
- 1 large onion, finely chopped
- 1 pound fresh green beans, trimmed
- 3 tablespoons tomato paste
- 1/2 teaspoon salt
- 2 tablespoons minced fresh parsley

Directions:

1.In a large skillet, heat the oil over medium-high heat. Add chopped onion; cook until tender and lightly browned, stirring occasionally.

2.Meanwhile, place green beans in a large saucepan; add water to cover. Bring to a boil. Cook, covered, for 5-7 minutes or until crisp-tender. Drain; add to onion. Stir in tomato paste and salt; heat through. Sprinkle with parsley.

Nutrition Info:
- 81 cal., 5g fat (1g sat. fat), 0 chol., 208mg sod., 9g carb. (4g sugars, 3g fiber), 2g pro.

Roasted Beets

Servings:4 | Cooking Time:60 Minutes

Ingredients:
- 1½ pounds beets, trimmed
- 1 tablespoon extra-virgin olive oil
- 1 tablespoon sherry vinegar
- 1 tablespoon minced fresh parsley
- Salt and pepper

Directions:

1.Adjust oven rack to middle position and heat oven to 400 degrees. Wrap beets individually in aluminum foil and place on rimmed baking sheet. Roast beets until skewer inserted into center meets little resistance (you will need to unwrap beets to test them), 45 to 60 minutes.

2.Remove beets from oven and slowly open foil packets (being careful of rising steam). When beets are cool enough to handle but still warm, gently rub off skins using paper towels.

3.Slice beets into ½-inch-thick wedges, then toss with oil, vinegar, parsley, and ¼ teaspoon salt. Season with pepper to taste and serve warm or at room temperature. (Beets can be refrigerated for up to 3 days; return to room temperature before serving.)

Nutrition Info:
- 80 cal., 3g fat (0g sag. fat), 0mg chol, 240mg sod., 11g carb (8g sugars, 3g fiber), 2g pro.

Broiled Eggplant With Basil

Servings:6 | Cooking Time:9 Minutes

Ingredients:
- 1½ pounds eggplant, sliced into ¼-inch-thick rounds
- Kosher salt and pepper
- 3 tablespoons extra-virgin olive oil
- 2 tablespoons chopped fresh basil

Directions:

1.Spread eggplant on paper towel–lined baking sheet, sprinkle both sides with 1½ teaspoons salt, and let sit for 9 minutes.

2.Adjust oven rack 4 inches from broiler element and heat broiler. Thoroughly pat eggplant dry with paper towels, arrange on aluminum foil–lined rimmed baking sheet in single layer, and brush both sides with oil. Broil eggplant until mahogany brown and lightly charred, about 4 minutes per side. Transfer eggplant to serving platter, season with pepper to taste, and sprinkle with basil. Serve.

Nutrition Info:
- 90 cal., 7g fat (1g sag. fat), 0mg chol, 140mg sod., 7g carb (4g sugars, 3g fiber), 1g pro.

Recipe

....

From the kicthen of ....

Serves .... Prep time .... Cook time ....

☐ Difficulty   ☐ Easy   ☐ Medium   ☐ Hard

Ingredient

Yummy!

....

....

....

....

....

Directions ....

....

....

....

....

....

....

Appendix A: Measurement Conversions

BASIC KITCHEN CONVERSIONS & EQUIVALENTS

DRY MEASUREMENTS CONVERSION CHART

3 TEASPOONS = 1 TABLESPOON = 1/16 CUP

6 TEASPOONS = 2 TABLESPOONS = 1/8 CUP

12 TEASPOONS = 4 TABLESPOONS = 1/4 CUP

24 TEASPOONS = 8 TABLESPOONS = 1/2 CUP

36 TEASPOONS = 12 TABLESPOONS = 3/4 CUP

48 TEASPOONS = 16 TABLESPOONS = 1 CUP

METRIC TO US COOKING CONVERSIONS

OVEN TEMPERATURES

120 °C = 250 °F

160 °C = 320 °F

180° C = 350 °F

205 °C = 400 °F

220 °C = 425 °F

LIQUID MEASUREMENTS CONVERSION CHART

8 FLUID OUNCES = 1 CUP = 1/2 PINT = 1/4 QUART

16 FLUID OUNCES = 2 CUPS = 1 PINT = 1/2 QUART

32 FLUID OUNCES = 4 CUPS = 2 PINTS = 1 QUART

= 1/4 GALLON

128 FLUID OUNCES = 16 CUPS = 8 PINTS = 4 QUARTS = 1 GALLON

BAKING IN GRAMS

1 CUP FLOUR = 140 GRAMS

1 CUP SUGAR = 150 GRAMS

1 CUP POWDERED SUGAR = 160 GRAMS

1 CUP HEAVY CREAM = 235 GRAMS

VOLUME

1 MILLILITER = 1/5 TEASPOON

5 ML = 1 TEASPOON

15 ML = 1 TABLESPOON

240 ML = 1 CUP OR 8 FLUID OUNCES

1 LITER = 34 FL. OUNCES

WEIGHT

1 GRAM = .035 OUNCES

100 GRAMS = 3.5 OUNCES

500 GRAMS = 1.1 POUNDS

1 KILOGRAM = 35 OUNCES

US TO METRIC COOKING CONVERSIONS

1/5 TSP = 1 ML

1 TSP = 5 ML

1 TBSP = 15 ML

1 FL OUNCE = 30 ML

1 CUP = 237 ML

1 PINT (2 CUPS) = 473 ML

1 QUART (4 CUPS) = .95 LITER

1 GALLON (16 CUPS) = 3.8 LITERS

1 OZ = 28 GRAMS

1 POUND = 454 GRAMS

BUTTER

1 CUP BUTTER = 2 STICKS = 8 OUNCES = 230 GRAMS = 8 TABLESPOONS

WHAT DOES 1 CUP EQUAL

1 CUP = 8 FLUID OUNCES

1 CUP = 16 TABLESPOONS

1 CUP = 48 TEASPOONS

1 CUP = 1/2 PINT

1 CUP = 1/4 QUART

1 CUP = 1/16 GALLON

1 CUP = 240 ML

BAKING PAN CONVERSIONS

1 CUP ALL-PURPOSE FLOUR = 4.5 OZ

1 CUP ROLLED OATS = 3 OZ 1 LARGE EGG = 1.7 OZ

1 CUP BUTTER = 8 OZ 1 CUP MILK = 8 OZ

1 CUP HEAVY CREAM = 8.4 OZ

1 CUP GRANULATED SUGAR = 7.1 OZ

1 CUP PACKED BROWN SUGAR = 7.75 OZ

1 CUP VEGETABLE OIL = 7.7 OZ

1 CUP UNSIFTED POWDERED SUGAR = 4.4 OZ

BAKING PAN CONVERSIONS

9-INCH ROUND CAKE PAN = 12 CUPS

10-INCH TUBE PAN =16 CUPS

11-INCH BUNDT PAN = 12 CUPS

9-INCH SPRINGFORM PAN = 10 CUPS

9 X 5 INCH LOAF PAN = 8 CUPS

9-INCH SQUARE PAN = 8 CUPS

Appendix B: Recipes Index

A

Apple Cinnamon Rollups   44
Asian Lettuce Wraps   46
Asian Snapper With Capers   63
Asparagus, Red Pepper, And Spinach Salad With Goat Cheese   22

B

Balsamic Zucchini Saute   68
Banana-pineapple Cream Pies   41
Basil Vegetable Strata   14
Beef En Cocotte With Mushrooms   33
Beets With Oranges And Walnuts   53
Bow Tie & Spinach Salad   26
Braised Pork Stew   33
Broiled Eggplant With Basil   69
Butternut Squash With Whole Grains   53

C

Caribbean Delight   46
Chard & Bacon Linguine   31
Cheese Manicotti   26
Cheesy Snack Mix   17
Chicken Enchiladas   48
Chicken, Mango & Blue Cheese Tortillas   18
Chickpea And Kale Soup   36
Chocolate-dipped Strawberry Meringue Roses   42
Creamy Curried Cauliflower Soup   38
Creamy Dill Sauce   62
Creamy Parmesan Polenta   57
Creamy Potato Soup With Green Onions   36
Crispy Fish & Chips   61
Crostini With Kalamata Tomato   18
Crunchy Pear And Cilantro Relish   67
Crunchy Tuna Wraps   64
Cumin-crusted Chicken Thighs With Cauliflower Couscous   49
Curried Chicken Skewers With Yogurt Dipping Sauce   13
Curried Tempeh With Cauliflower And Peas   28

D

Dill-marinated Broccoli   23
Double-duty Banana Pancakes   13

F

Farro Bowl With Tofu, Mushrooms, And Spinach   29
Fennel, Apple, And Chicken Chopped Salad   23
Fresh Lemon Roasted Brussels Sprouts   66
Frittata With Spinach, Bell Pepper, And Basil   12
Fusilli With Skillet-roasted Cauliflower, Garlic, And Walnuts   56
Fusilli With Zucchini, Tomatoes, And Pine Nuts   58

G

Garlic-chicken And Wild Rice Soup   39
Gorgonzola Polenta Bites   16
Grapefruit-zested Pork   34
Grilled Chicken Kebabs With Tomato-feta Salad   47

H

Herbed Potato Packet   66
Honey-yogurt Berry Salad   11

I

Italian Cabbage Soup   52

L

Lemon-herb Cod Fillets With Garlic Potatoes   63

M

Maple Apple Baked Oatmeal   12
Mexican-style Spaghetti Squash Casserole   27
Mocha Pumpkin Seeds   17
Moroccan-style Carrot Salad   21
Mushroom And Wheat Berry Soup   39
Mustard Vinaigrette With Lemon And Parsley   61

N

No-fuss Banana Ice Cream   42

O

Omega-3 Granola   11
Oven-fried Chicken Drumsticks   47
Oven-roasted Salmon   63

P

Peaches, Blackberries, And Strawberries With Basil And Pepper   44
Pineapple Breeze Torte   41
Pomegranate And Nut Chocolate Clusters   43
Porcini-marsala Pan Sauce   31
Pork Loin With Fennel, Oranges, And Olives   54
Pumpkin Turkey Chili   38

R

Radish, Orange, And Avocado Chopped Salad   21
Rainbow Veggie Salad   22
Raisin & Hummus Pita Wedges   19
Roasted Asparagus   68
Roasted Beets   69

S

Salmon Dill Soup   37
Sassy Salsa Meat Loaves   32
Saucy Spiced Pears   43
Sausage-egg Burritos   14
Sautéed Swiss Chard With Garlic   67
Shrimp Avocado Salad   64
Shrimp Pad Thai Soup   37
Slow Cooker Mushroom Chicken & Peas   51
Spaghetti And Meatballs   59
Spaghetti Squash With Garlic And Parmesan   68
Spaghetti With Spinach, Beans, Tomatoes, And Garlic Chips   57
Spiced Pork Tenderloin With Carrots And Radishes   51
Spicy Tomato Pork Chops   34
Spinach Salad With Carrots, Oranges, And Sesame   24
Stewed Beef And Ale   34
Stewed Chickpeas With Eggplant And Tomatoes   27
Sweet Onion & Red Bell Pepper Topping   53
Sweet Peanut Buttery Dip   16
Sweet Sherry'd Pork Tenderloin   32

T

Taco-spiced Rice   56
Tangy Sweet Carrot Pepper Salad   24
Tasty Lentil Tacos   29
Teriyaki Beef Stew   52
Thai-style Red Curry With Cauliflower   28
Tomato-onion Green Beans   69
Tuna Salad Stuffed Eggs   19
Turkey Chili   54
Turkey Cutlets With Barley And Broccoli   49
Turkey Sausage Zucchini Boats   48
Two-sauce Cajun Fish   62

W

Warm Farro With Fennel And Parmesan   59
Warm Farro With Mushrooms And Thyme   58
Warm Figs With Goat Cheese And Honey   43
Wicked Deviled Eggs   18

Z

Zesty Citrus Melon   23

Made in the USA
Las Vegas, NV
06 November 2023